CRANIOFACIAL DEVELOPMENT

Geoffrey H. Sperber
BSc (Hons), BDS, MS, PhD, FICD
Professor Emeritus
Faculty of Medicine and Dentistry
University of Alberta
Edmonton, Alberta

Illustrations by Jackie Wald
BC Decker Inc

CD-ROM computer images by Geoffrey D. Guttmann, PhD,
and Steven M. Sperber, MSc

2001
BC Decker Inc
Hamilton • London

BC Decker Inc
20 Hughson Street South
P.O. Box 620, L.C.D. 1
Hamilton, Ontario L8N 3K7
Tel: 905-522-7017; 1-800-568-7281
Fax: 905-522-7839
E-mail: info@bcdecker.com
Website: www.bcdecker.com

00 01 02 03 / PC / 9 8 7 6 5 4 3 2 1

ISBN 1-55009-127-1

Printed in Canada

Sales and Distribution

United States
B.C. Decker Inc.
P.O. Box 785
Lewiston, NY 14092-0785
Tel: 905-522-7017 / 1-800-568-7281
Fax: 905-522-7839
E-mail: info@bcdecker.com
Website: www.bcdecker.com

Canada
B.C. Decker Inc.
20 Hughson Street South
P.O. Box 620, L.C.D. 1
Hamilton, Ontario L8N 3K7
Tel: 905-522-7017 / 1-800-568-7281
Fax: 905-522-7839
E-mail: info@bcdecker.com
Website: www.bcdecker.com

Japan
Igaku-Shoin Ltd.
Foreign Publications Department
3-24-17 Hongo
Bunkyo-ku,Tokyo, Japan 113-8719
Tel: 3 3817 5680
Fax: 3 3815 6776
E-mail: fd@igaku.shoin.co.jp

Foreign Rights
John Scott & Company
International Publishers' Agency
P.O. Box 878
Kimberton, PA 19442
Tel: 610-827-1640
Fax: 610-827-1671

U.K., Europe, Scandinavia, Middle East
Harcourt Publishers Limited
Customer Service Department
Foots Cray High Street
Sidcup, Kent
DA14 5HP, UK
Tel: 44 (0) 208 308 5760
Fax: 44 (0) 181 308 5702
E-mail: cservice@harcourt_brace.com

Australia
Harcourt Australia Pty. Limited
Customer Service Department
STM Division, Locked Bag 16
St. Peters, New South Wales, 2044
Australia
Tel: 02 9517-8999
Fax: 02 9517-2249
e-mail: stmp@harcourt.com.au
website: www.harcourt.com.au

Singapore, Malaysia, Thailand, Philippines,
Indonesia, Vietnam, Pacific Rim
Harcourt Asia Pte Limited
583 Orchard Road
#09/01, Forum
Singapore 238884
Tel: 65-737-3593
Fax: 65-753-2145

Front Cover

Three dimensional computer-reconstructed head of a sectioned human 55-day-old post conception fetus. The brain and eyes are rendered in blue; the cartilages in white; the oronasopharynx in green; the inner ear in yellow; the notochord in purple; the trigeminal ganglion in brown; the arteries in red; the skin outline is translucent. (Courtesy of S. M. Sperber)

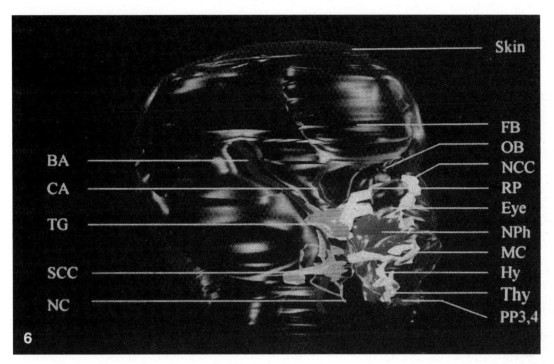

BA:	Basilar artery (red)	MC:	Meckel's cartilage (white)
CA:	Carotid artery (red)	Hy:	Hyoid cartilage (white)
FB:	Forebrain (blue)	Thy:	Thyroid cartilage (white)
OB:	Olfactory bulbs (blue)	PP3.4	Third and fourth pharyngeal
NCC:	Nasal capsule cartilage (white)		pouches (green)
RP:	Rathke's pouch (green)	TG:	Trigeminal ganglion (brown)
NPh:	Nasopharynx (green)	SCC:	Semicircular canals (yellow)
NC:	Notochord (purple)		

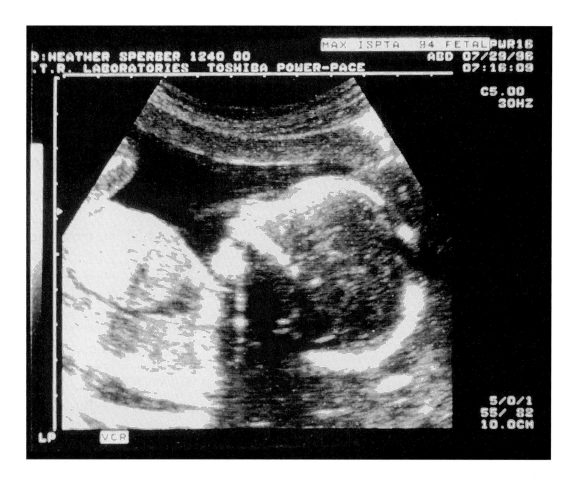

Ultrasonography has converted embryology and fetology from esoteric basic sciences into clinically relevant disciplines by making the fetus a potential patient. An ultrasonograph of the head and thorax of a normal 18-week-old fetus in utero.

FOREWORD

The last few decades of the twentieth century have brought numerous advances, in both concepts and technology, into the biomedical disciplines. Indeed, no branch of biology—from paleoanthropology to the neurosciences, from cell biology to ontogeny—has been untouched by the new approaches; this is certainly true in regard to the fields of embryology and developmental anatomy.

The old science of embryology was largely a descriptive account of the kaleidoscope of changes from the fertilized ovum through the stages of the zygote, embryo, and fetus to the full-term baby. When I was a student, embryology seemed to be a largely theoretic account of small relevance to the medical and dental professions. Except for when it was well taught and its clinical relevance was brought to the fore, students tended to suffer from just another burden. Even though the fascinating field of experimental embryology had been in existence for over a century, it seldom found its way into the syllabus for developmental studies taught to medical and dental students. More is the pity, for those students would have found much to excite their sense of wonderment. At the same time, they would have been brought closer to an understanding of how it sometimes happens that the train of development is shunted from the main railroad onto a sidetrack leading to variations, anomalies, and more dramatically, congenital malformations. All of these outcomes of shunted development are clinically relevant. It has become possible—through amniocentesis, cell biology, and DNA sequencing—to diagnose such maldevelopments earlier and earlier in fetal life. At its simplest, this may help plan the handling of a pregnancy; but it may also make intrauterine therapy possible. So, not only diagnosis but treatment is being applied in selected cases in which human mothers are suspected to be carrying defective or abnormal fetuses.

Open heart surgery was introduced when Alfred Blalock and Helen Taussig devised an operation to correct congenital malformations of the heart. Suddenly, it became desperately important for clinicians to learn about the normal embryonic development of the heart to understand its abnormal development better. What had previously required a rather tedious effort to memorize the embryonic development of the heart in the hope that this might better aid the student's understanding of the finished product—the healthy heart—now assumed an obvious relevance for the diagnosis and treatment of congenital malformations. Heart surgeons began queueing up to gain admission to anatomy departments to learn the basics of cardiac embryology!

If that was the situation in the third quarter of the twentieth century, even greater advances were chalked up in the final quarter. The understanding of developmental phenomena became greatly enhanced, and with it, the clinical, diagnostic, and therapeutic potential. The use of such new technical marvels as ultrasonography, DNA sequencing following amniocentesis, and many other imaging procedures all conspired to produce a new dimension in developmental studies. How far we have traveled since Leonardo da Vinci measured a series of human embryos and fetuses of different ages 500 years ago! As we stand on the threshold of a new century and a new millennium for some members of the human species, who can say how much more we may comprehend by the end of the next 500 years? But let us not lift our eyes so far into the future. What will be the state of our knowledge of the human body, its evolution, and its ontogeny by the next 50 years? I shall not be here to witness these new miracles, but even if I were to be here, I am sure I would not understand how they worked. Many students of today who read this book will certainly be alive, and I am confident that among them will be some of the architects of the New Developmental Biology.

I have mentioned the congenital malformations of the heart; this was simply because the heart was the first internal organ to be operated on to correct developmental anomalies. Perhaps no part of the body is more liable to developmental deviations, more amenable to embryologic analysis, and more a part of everyday clinical practice than the head and neck. Most organs of the body are concealed below the surface; but we are not ashamed to show our teeth when we smile or eat or speak—or yawn or sneeze. Faces and teeth and jaws are on or close to the surface of the head; we should know more about them than about any parts that modesty or our bodily structure conceal.

Dr. Geoffrey Sperber realized this nearly 30 years ago when he produced his admirable little book titled *Craniofacial Embryology*. Through four editions and several translations, that book took the message to thousands of undergraduate and graduate students and lecturers all over the world. Now, with these new approaches knocking on the door, a new book has become necessary, incorporating the new concepts of development and the new techniques for elucidating it. Professor Sperber takes us by the hand and shows us how to understand cleft palates, underdeveloped jaws, too many (or too few) teeth, and very large tongues or very small mouths: they are the end results of lines of development different in one or another respect from the usual pathways. He enables us to appreciate that the developmental approach is a vital key to the mastery of the aberrant as well as the normal.

Professor Sperber's dual background in dentistry and anatomy has made him well placed to achieve his objective. His meticulous attention to detail, coupled with a clear appreciation of the signposts leading through the maze of items and processes, has enabled him to give us an extremely useful text, of a pioneering kind.

This is a book from which undergraduate and graduate students of dentistry, oral medicine, orthodontics, head and neck surgery, dental anatomy, speech pathology, and anthropology should benefit immensely.

To you who read this book, I hope you will be not only enlightened but delighted. Forget the stricture of Benjamin Disraeli that "Books are fatal: they are the curse of the human race." Rather, see this book as a guide to the perplexed and a source of truth—and revel in it to get the most out of it. Remember what Confucius said: "Those who know the truth are not equal to those who love it, nor those who love it to those who delight in it." I wish all the readers of this work many hours of joy, for nothing makes the task of learning easier and more palatable than to read without tears, to chew over a subject, and to enjoy the taste.

Phillip V. Tobias, DSc, PhD, MB BCh, FRS, FRCP

ACKNOWLEDGEMENTS

This book could not have been accomplished without the inspiration and unstinting assistance of numerous colleagues and helpers to whom I am deeply indebted. Most particularly do I wish to express my special gratitude to Mrs. Anne-Marie McLean whose patience and cheerfulness in typing and retyping several drafts of the text with meticulous concern for accuracy ensured a fault-free typescript delivered to the publisher. Many of the diagrams appearing in the predecessor "Craniofacial Embryology", drawn by Dr. Anthony M. MacIsaac have been reproduced, and more diagrams by Mrs. Jackie Wald have been added.

My thanks go to the authors and publishers of diagrams and photographs, acknowledged in the captions, who so generously gave me permission to reproduce their copyright material in this work. The copyright permissions granted by Saunders, Springer, Lippincott-Raven, and Butterworth-Heinemann are gratefully acknowledged.

My appreciation is extended to Professor Emeritus Phillip V. Tobias for providing the Foreword, to Dr. Emile Rossouw for contributing a section on cephalometrics, and to Professor W.H. Arnold, Steven Sperber, and Dr. Geoffrey Guttmann for producing computer-created 3-D images of sectioned embryos for the CD-ROM.

The encouragement by Paul Donnelly and Brian Decker to produce this publication is acknowledged in its fulfilment.

My affectionate thanks to my wife, Robyn, my daughters Heather and Jacqueline and their families, and my inspiring son Steven for their forgiving of my time spent in the preparation of this work.

GHS

PREFACE

The genesis of this book can be traced to the four editions of its predecessor "Craniofacial Embryology" that has enlightened students in the intricacies of development of the cephalic region for over a quarter of a century. The translation of these previous works into Japanese, German, and Indonesian editions indicates widespread interest in utilizing this text in many parts of the world.

Replacement of that now outdated text is necessitated by the new technologies that have revealed deeper insights into the mechanisms of embryogenesis. The Human Genome Project, now completed, and the explosion of molecular biological knowledge are expanding exponentially our understanding of the development and maldevelopment of the human organism. Moreover, the realm of the once esoteric study of embryology has been vaulted into clinical conscience now that in vitro fertilization, choronic villus sampling, amniocentesis and prenatal ultrasonography and even prenatal fetal surgery are becoming part of clinical practice (Frontispiece). All these aforementioned procedures require an intimate knowledge of the different stages of development, to which this book is dedicated.

The increasing sophistication of prenatal imaging techniques is revealing ever - earlier stages of fetal formation, and significantly, malformation, that may require intervention. To that end, increased emphasis has been placed on anomalous development, allowing for informed decision - making on possible reparative or "genetically engineered" therapy. The combining of "basic science" embryology and fetology with its consequences on clinical practice is one of the aims of this text in breaking barriers between "scientists" and "clinicians" in advancing our understanding the causes, prognosis, and treatments of dysmorphology that is becoming an extensive component of modern medicine and its allied professions.

The advent of computer technology has enabled the portrayal of developmental phenomena as three-dimensional model images in sequential depictions of changes proceeding in the fourth dimension of time. This "morphing" technique is a powerful adjunct to gaining understanding of the complexities of rapidly changing tissues, organs, and relationships occurring during embryogenesis. Some of these animated sequences have been added as an electronic adjunct to the text in the accompanying CD-ROM.

It is hoped that the disparate disciplines of anatomy, embryology, syndromology, plastic and orofacial surgery, otolaryngology, orthodontics, pediatrics, dentistry, speech pathology, and associated health care fields will find a melding of their diverse interests in the common objective of understanding and providing diagnosis, prognosis, prevention, and cure of the disparities of development of the craniofacial complex. To this purpose is this book committed.

GHS
October 2000

SECTION I

GENERAL EMBRYOLOGY

SECTION II

CRANIOFACIAL DEVELOPMENT

SECTION I

GENERAL EMBRYOLOGY

1 MECHANISMS OF EMBRYOLOGY

There must be a beginning of any great matter, but the continuing unto the end until it be thoroughly finished, yields the true glory.

Sir Francis Drake, 1587

Unraveling the incredibly complex combination of molecular events that constitute the creation of a human embryo is a form of ultradissection at biochemical, cellular, organismic and systemic levels at different stages of development. The reconstitution of these unraveled discrete events provides a basis for understanding the mechanisms of embryogenesis.

The new reproductive technologic revolution instigated by laboratory in vitro fertilization (versus the old-fashioned in vivo method of fertilization) has sparked enormous advances in the understanding of the cascade of reactions initiated by the conjunction of viable spermatozoa with an ovum, whether it be abnormally in a petri dish or normally in the oviduct. Insights into developmental phenomena are dependent on a knowledge of genetics, gene expression, receptor mechanisms, signal transduction, and the differentiation of the totipotential stem cells into the different cell types that form tissues, organs, and systems. Understanding these phenomena is changing embryology from a descriptive science into a predictive science with the potential for control of embryologic mechanisms.

GENETICS

The concept of a gene as director of development in conjunction with environmental influences needs to be understood in different contexts. The classical concept of a gene as a unit of *recombination* refers to a single deoxyribonucleic acid (DNA) nucleotide base pair, whereas consideration of a gene as a unit of *mutation* varies biochemically from a single base pair to hundreds of nucleotide base pairs. The embryologically significant gene as a unit of *function* is a sequence of hundreds or thousands of nucleotides that specify the sequence of amino acids that make up the primary structure of a polypeptide chain. These polypeptide chains constitute the proteins that provide the cells that form the tissues that create the organs of a developing embryo. Functionally, genes are conceived as structural, operator, or regulatory genes (Fig. 1–1).

The term *genome* refers to the array of genes (as defined above) in a complete haploid set of chromosomes that is expressed as the functional *genotype* in development, and that, in combination with environmental influences, results in formation of the *phenotype*, the physical and behavioral traits of an organism. The human genome,* having been mapped by the Human Genome

---

*The size of the genome is independent of its genetic information. A single-cell amoeba has a genome of > 200,000 megabases; the human genome has about 3,000 megabases.

Project, is believed to contain 3×10^9 (3 billion) nucleotide bases that constitute a variably estimated 35,000 to 120,000 genes. The identification and mapping of these genes, with specific positions (loci) on the chromosomes and with their nomenclature, is a task of increasing difficulty that is being standardized by the establishment of computerized Web sites that are continually updated as new data become available.

Regulation of the genetic program underlying cell differentiation and morphogenesis is due to differential gene activity. Cell fates, mitotic and apoptopic (cell death) activity, migratory patterns, and metabolic states are determined by genes turning on and off at critical times. There is a high degree of order in the genetic program, bolstered by redundancy and overlapping of expression patterns to guide morphogenesis. Intervention in developmental programs forms the basis of experimental embryology and offers the potential for "genetic engineering" of deleterious or advantageous mutations. The rapid rate of cell division in the fetus may allow in utero vectored gene therapy for previously diagnosed mutations to correct genetic defects. Epigenesis describes the phenomena occurring after genetic determination.

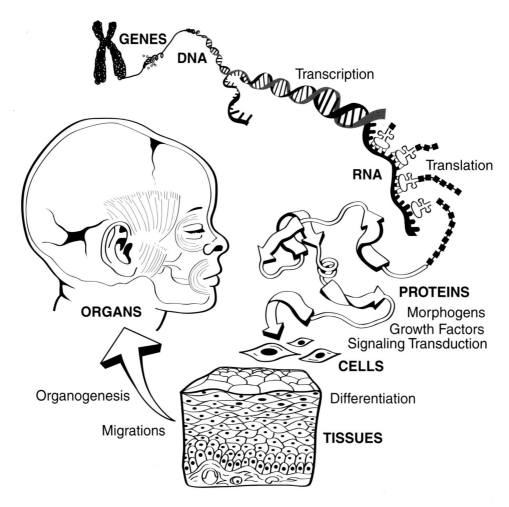

Figure 1–1 Schematic synopsis of the sequence of development from genes to fetus (DNA = deoxyribonucleic acid; RNA = ribonucleic acid).

Genes control the synthesis of proteins, of which some 200,000 to 300,000 varieties have been identified, to create 200 or so cell types that proliferate into approximately 10^{14} cells, forming 220 named structures in an average human adult. The longevity and proliferation of differentiated cells is also genetically determined in three broad categories:

1. Continuous mitotics (with short life spans)—for example, epithelia
2. Intermittent mitotics—for example, liver cells (hepatocytes)
3. Postmitotics (with long life spans)—for example, neurons.

SIGNAL TRANSDUCTION

Intercellular communication plays a major role in controlling development. Transcription factors regulate the identity and patterning of embryonic structures and the development of individual organs. Organizing centers are created that serve as the source of signals that guide the patterning of organs and ultimately of the whole embryo. A signaling center or node (eg, Hensen's node) is a cell group that regulates the behavior of surrounding cells by producing positive and negative intercellular signaling molecules. Genes encode extracellular matrix proteins, cell adhesion molecules, and cytoplasmic signaling pathway components. An ever increasing number of signaling factors influencing development are being identified (Table 1–1).

Growth factors stimulate cell proliferation and differentiation by acting through specific receptors on responsive cells. Most of these growth factors are present and active throughout life, assuming different roles at different times and places but displaying remarkable conservation of functional mechanisms. Thus, growth factors play analagous roles in embryogenesis, in the immune system, and during inflammation and wound repair. This has given rise to the concept of "ontogenetic inflammation," by which normal embryonic development may act as a prototype for inflammation and healing that regulates homeostasis in the adult. Diffusion of these molecules and differential concentration gradients creates fields of influence, determining differentiation patterns that form fate maps. After a signaling center has fulfilled its task, it gradually disappears.

Patterning of the development of regions, organs, and systems is controlled by genes expressed as growth factor signaling molecules. The early development of a *primitive streak* (a rapidly proliferating elongating mass of cells in the embryonic germ disk) demarcates the initial distinction of embryonic tissues. A gene, Lim–1, is essential for the organization of the primitive streak and for the development of the entire head. After the initial differentiation of the primary germ layers by reciprocal interactions between cells and tissues, segmentation is a feature of early embryogenesis. Such segmentation is manifested in the ectodermal neural tube by four regions: forebrain, midbrain, hindbrain, and spinal cord, with the hindbrain further segmented into seven or eight rhombomeres. Paraxial mesoderm is segmented cranially into seven swellings termed *somitomeres* and caudally into 38 to 42 somites. The six pharyngeal arches are a third visibly segmented set of tissues (Fig. 1–2). Under the

TABLE 1–1 Signaling and Growth Factors

Factor	Abbreviation	Derivation	Action
Bone morphogenetic proteins	BMPs (1-8)	Pharyngeal arches; frontonasal mass	Mesoderm induction; Dorso-ventral organizer; Skeletogenesis; Neurogenesis
Brain-derived neurotrophic factor	BDNF	Neural tube	Stimulates dorsal root ganglia anlagen
Distal-less	Dlx	Genome	Transcriptional activator
Epidermal growth factor	EGF	Various organs; salivary glands	Stimulates proliferation and differentiation of many cell types
Fibroblastic growth factors (1-19)	FGFs	Various organs and organizing centers	Neural and mesoderm induction. Stimulates proliferation of fibroblasts, endothelium, myoblasts, osteoblasts
Hepatocyte growth factor	HGF	Pharyngeal arches	Cranial motor axon growth; Angiogenesis
Homeodomain proteins	Hox-a,Hox-b, Pax, Dlx	Genome	Craniocaudal and Dorsoventral patterning
Insulin-like growth factors 1 and 2	IGF-1 IGF-2	Sympathetic chain ganglia	Stimulates proliferation of fat and connective tissues and metabolism
Interleukin-2, Interleukin-3, Interleukin-4	IL-2 IL-3, IL-4	White blood cells	Stimulates proliferation of T-lymphocytes; Hematopoietic growth-factor; B-cell growth factor
Lymphoid enhancer factor 1	Lef1	Neural crest; Mesencephalon	Regulates epithelial-mesenchymal interactions
Nerve growth factor	NGF	Various organs	Promotes axon growth and neuron survival
Platelet-derived growth factor	PDGF	Platelets	Stimulates proliferation of fibroblasts, neurons, smooth muscle cells and neuroglia
Sonic hedgehog	Shh	Various organs	Neural plate and Craniocaudal patterning, Chondrogenesis
Transcriptional factors	TFs	Intermediate gene in mesoderm induction casade	Stimulates transcription of actin gene
Transforming growth factor-α	TGF-α	Various organs	Promotes differentiation of certain cells
Transforming growth factor-β (Activin A, Activin B)	TGF-β	Various organs	Mesoderm induction; Potentiates or inhibits responses to other growth factors
Vascular endothelial growth factor	VEGF	Smooth muscle cells	Stimulates angiogenesis
Wingless	Wnt	Genome	Pattern formation; organizer

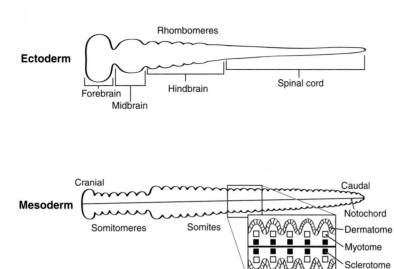

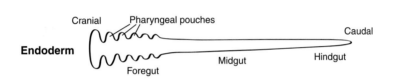

Figure 1–2 Schematic depiction of segmentation in early embryogenesis in the primary germ layers.

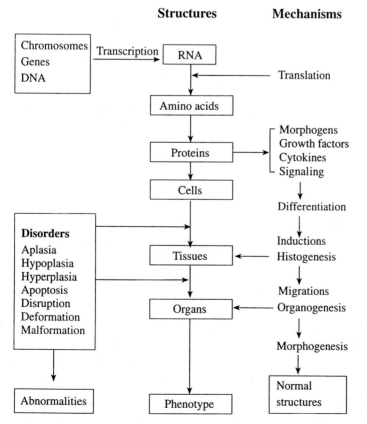

Figure 1–3 Flow chart of developmental phenomena. DNA, deoxyribonucleic acid; RNA, ribonucleic acid. (Reproduced with permission from Sperber GH. Ann Acad Med Singapore 1999;28:708–13.)

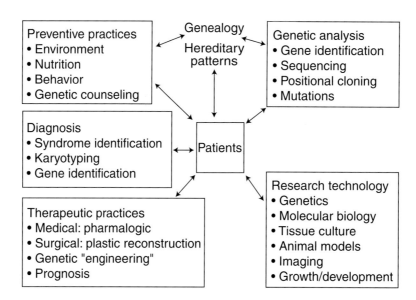

Figure 1–4 Schema for patient-centered procedures. (Reproduced with permission from Sperber GH. Ann Acad Med Singapore 1999; 28:708–13.)

control of regulatory homeobox genes (Hoxa-1, Hoxa-2, Hoxb-1, Hoxb-3, Hoxb-4, sonic hedgehog [SHH], Krox-20, patched [Ptc], paired box, [Pax1.9]), the segmented tissues are integrated into morphologically identifiable structures.

The mapping of genetic loci and the identification of mutant genes related to congenital defects and clinical syndromes are revealing the mechanisms of morphogenesis. The etiology and embryopathogenesis of a number of diverse anomalies of development are being traced to a common molecular basis. The recognition of growth and signaling factors (intercellular mediators) and their receptors (specific binding agents) and the expression domains of genes is providing insights into the mechanisms of normal and anomalous development (Fig. 1–3).

The developmental ontogeny of the craniofacial odontostomatognathic complex depends primarily on the following three elements:

1. Genetic factors: inherited genotype; expression of genetic mechanisms
2. Environmental factors: nutritional and biochemical interactions; physical phenomena—temperature, pressures, hydration, etc.
3. Functional factors: extrinsic and intrinsic forces of muscle actions, space-occupying cavities and organs, growth expansion, and atrophic attenuation

The central theme of patient care, around which rotate therapists and researchers, provides interactive feedback for insights into developmental phenomena and their aberrations (Fig. 1–4).

Selected Bibliography

Anonymous. Research advances in prenatal craniofacial development. In honor of Robert M. Pratt. Proceedings of an international congress. North Carolina, 1988. J Craniofac Genet Dev Biol 1991;11:181–378.

Avery J. Oral development and histology. 3rd ed. New York: Thieme Medical Publishers; 2001.

Carlson BM. Human embryology and developmental biology. 2nd ed. St. Louis: Mosby Yearbook; 1999.

Francis-West P, Ladher R, Barlow A, Graveson A. Signaling interactions during facial development. Mech Dev 1998;75:3–28.

Gerhart J. Signaling pathways in development. Teratology 1999;60:226–39.

Greene RM. Signal transduction during craniofacial development. Crit Rev Toxicol 1989;20:137–52.

Greene RM, Pisano MM. Pathways to transcription. Teratology 2000;62:10–3.

Gullberg D, Ekblom P. Extracellular matrix and its receptors during development. Int J Dev Biol 1995;39:845–54.

Hall BK. Germ layers and the germ layer theory revisited. Evol Biol 1998; 30:121–86.

Hall BK. Evolutionary issues in craniofacial biology. Cleft Palate J 1990;27:95–100.

Hart TC, Marazita ML, Wright JT. The impact of molecular genetics on oral health paradigms. Crit Rev Oral Biol Med 2000;11:26–56.

Hogan BL, Blessing M, Winnier GE, et al. Growth factors in development: the role of TGF-beta related polypeptide signaling molecules in embryogenesis. Dev Suppl 1994;53–60.

Howe AM, Webster WS. Vitamin K—its essential role in craniofacial development. A review of the literature regarding vitamin K and craniofacial development. Aust Dent J 1994;39:88–92.

Hunt P, Clarke JDW, Buxton P, et al. Segmentation crest prespecification and the control of facial form. Eur J Oral Sci 1998;106 Suppl:12–18.

Kalyani AJ, Rao MS. Cell lineage in the developing neural tube. Biochem Cell Biol 1998;76:1051–68.

Kerrigan JJ, McGill JT, Davies JA, et al. The role of cell adhesion molecules in craniofacial development. J Coll Surg Edinb 1998;43:223–9.

Larsen WJ . Human embryology. 2nd ed. New York: Churchill Livingstone; 1997.

Le Douarin NM, Kalcheim C. The neural crest. 2nd ed. New York: Cambridge University Press; 1999.

Moiseiwitsch JRD. The role of serotonin and neurotransmitters during craniofacial development. Crit Rev Oral Biol Med 2000;11:230–9.

Moore KL. The developing human: clinically orientated embryology. 6th ed. Philadelphia: W.B. Saunders; 1998.

Morriss-Kay GM, Sokolova N. Embryonic development and pattern formation. FASEB J 1996;10:961–8.

Munne S, Cohen J. Chromosome abnormalities in human embryos. Hum Reprod Update 1998;4:842–55.

Opitz JM. Blastogenesis and the "primary field" in human development. Birth Defects Orig Artic Ser 1993;29:3–37.

Portin P. The concept of the gene: short history and present status. Q Rev Biol 1993;68:173–223.

Pirinen S. Genetic craniofacial aberrations. Acta Odontol Scand1998;56:356–9.

Rédei GP. Genetics manual. Singapore: World Scientific Pub. Co.; 1998.

Richman JM, Rowe A, Brickell PM. Signals involved in patterning and morphogenesis of the embryonic face. Prog Clin Biol Res 1991;373:117–31.

Rossel M, Capecchi MR. Mice mutant for both hoxa1 and hoxb1 show extensive remodeling of the hindbrain and defects in craniofacial development. Development 1999;126:5027–40.

Sandy JR. Signal transduction. Br J Orthod 1998;25:269–74.

Sela-Donenfeld D, Kalcheim C. Regulation of the onset of neural crest migration by coordinated activity of BMP4 and Noggin in the dorsal neural tube. Development 1999;126:4749–62.

Sharpe PT. Homeobox genes and orofacial development. Connect Tissue Res 1995;32:17–25.

Shuler CF. Programmed cell death and cell transformation in craniofacial development. Crit Rev Oral Biol Med 1995;6:202–17.

Sperber GH. First year of life: prenatal craniofacial development. Cleft Palate Craniofac J 1992;29:109–11.

Sperber GH. Current concepts in embryonic craniofacial development. Crit Rev Oral Biol Med 1992;4:67–72.

Sperber GH, Machin GA. The enigma of cephalogenesis. Cleft Palate Craniofac J 1994;31:91–6.

Stewart CL, Cullinan FB. Preimplantation development of the mammalian embryo and its regulation by growth factors. Dev Genet 1997;21:91–101.

Strachan T, Abitbol M, Davidson D, Beckmann JS. A new dimension for the human genome project: towards comprehensive expression maps. Nat Genet 1997;16:126–32.

Thesleff I. The genetic basis of normal and abnormal craniofacial development. Acta Odontal Scand 1998;56:321–5.

Wood R, editor. Genetic nomenclature guide with information on websites. Cambridge (UK): Elsevier Trends Journals; 1998.

Wozney JM. The bone morphogenetic protein family: multifunctional cellular regulators in the embryo and adult. Eur J Sci 1998;106:160–6.

Young E, Schneider RA, Hu D, Helms JA. Genetic and teratogenic approaches to craniofacial development. Crit Rev Oral Biol Med 2000;11:304–17.

Web Sites

HUGO Gene Nomenclature Committee. 2000 July 5 [accessed 2000 July 25]. URL: http://www.gene.ucl.ac.uk/nomenclature

Human Genome Resources; Genomes guide. 2000 Jan 27 [accessed 2000 July 25]. URL:http://www.ncbi.nlm.nih.gov/genome/guide

2 EARLY EMBRYONIC DEVELOPMENT

Over the structure of the cell rises the structure of plants and animals, which exhibit the yet more complicated, elaborate combinations of millions and billions of cells coordinated and differentiated in the most extremely different way.

Oscar Hertwig

The mating of male and female gametes in the maternal uterine tube initiates the development of a zygote—the first identification of an individual. The union of the haploid number of chromosomes (23) of each gamete confers the hereditary material of each parent upon the newly established diploid number of chromosomes (46) of the zygote. All the inherited characteristics of an individual and its sex are thereby established at the time of union of the gametes. The single totipotential cell (approximately 140 μm in diameter) resulting from the union very soon commences mitotic division to produce a rapidly increasing number of smaller cells, so that the 16-cell stage, known as the morula, is not much larger than the initial zygote. These cells of the early zygote reveal no significant outward differences of form. However, the chromosomes of these cells must necessarily contain the potential for differentiation of subsequent cell generations into the variety of cell forms that later constitute the different tissues of the body. The genetic material contained in the reconstituted diploid number of 46 chromosomes of the initial zygote cell is identical, by replication, to that contained in its progeny. The activity of this replicated genetic material varies as the subsequent cell generations depart from the archetype "primitive" cell. Different parts of the genetic material are active at different stages of development. Proliferation of the cells of the zygote allows the expression of their potential for differentiation into the great variety of cell types that constitute the different tissues of the body. The differentiation of these early pluripotential cells into specialized forms depends on genetic, cytoplasmic, and environmental factors that act at critical times during cell proliferation and growth.

DIFFERENTIATION

The transformation of the ovum into a full-fledged organism (during which there is an orderly diversification of the proliferating cells of the morula) is the result of selective activation and repression of the diploid set of genes carried in each cell. Which one of a pair of gene alleles contained in the diploid set of autosomal chromosomes is expressed depends on their similarity (homozygosity) or dissimilarity (heterozygosity). In the latter case, the degree of dominance or recessiveness of each allele of the pair determines the phenotypic expression of the gene. The expression of the traits governed by genes on the pair of nonautosomal or sex chromosomes is somewhat different. In females, there is inactivation of one of the two X chromosomes and failure of expression of its genes (the Lyon hypothesis). In males, the presence of the Y chromosome and only a single X chromosome accounts for the sex linkage of certain inherited traits.

A programmed sequence of development, known as epigenesis, is dependent on determination that restricts multipotentiality and causes differentiation of proliferating cells. These developmental events result from continuous interactions between cells and their microenvironments. As a consequence of differentiation, new varieties of cell types and tissues develop that interact with one another by induction (a morphogenetic effect by organizers), producing an increasingly complex organism. Induction alters the developmental course of responsive tissues (whose capacity to react is termed competence) to produce the different tissues from which organs and systems arise. Inductive interactions may take place in several ways in different tissues. Interactions may occur by direct cellular contact or may be mediated by diffusible agents or even by inductors enclosed in vesicles. The mechanisms involved in these processes include gene activation and inactivation, protein translation mechanics, varying cell membrane selectivities, intercellular adhesions and repulsions, and cell migrations that produce precise cell positioning. As microenvironments activate or inhibit mechanisms leading to cellular diversification, cell position and adhesion are key factors in early morphogenesis. All these events are critically timed and are under hormonal, metabolic, and nutritional influences. The biochemical foundations of these complex functions and the nature and manner of operation of their controlling factors, which are being widely explored, are among the central challenges of contemporary biology. The identification of morphogens (determining differentiation) and teratogens (disturbing normal morphogenesis) is the current focus of developmental biologists.

Units of cells and tissues form morphogenetic fields, which follow genetic and epigenetic phases of morphogenesis. Fields are susceptible to alteration by the interplay of genetic and environmental factors. The peak period of morphogenesis of a developmental field is a critical period of sensitivity to environmental and teratogenic disturbances. A compendium of manifold biochemical reactions leads to cytodifferentiation and histodifferentiation, resulting in the formation of epithelial and mesenchymal tissues that acquire a specialized structure and function (Fig. 2–1). Epithelial-mesenchymal interactions that provide for reciprocal cell differentiation are essential to organogenesis, that is, the production of organs and systems (Fig. 2–2).

The entire group of the above processes is marvelously integrated to form the external and internal configuration of the embryo, constituting morphogenesis, the process of development of form and size that determines the morphology of organs, systems, and the entire body. Not only are mitosis and cell growth essential for embryonic development, but paradoxically, even cell death—genetically and hormonally controlled—forms a significant part of normal embryogenesis. By means of programmed cell death, tissues and organs useful only during embryonic life are eliminated along with phylogenetic vestiges developed during ontogeny.

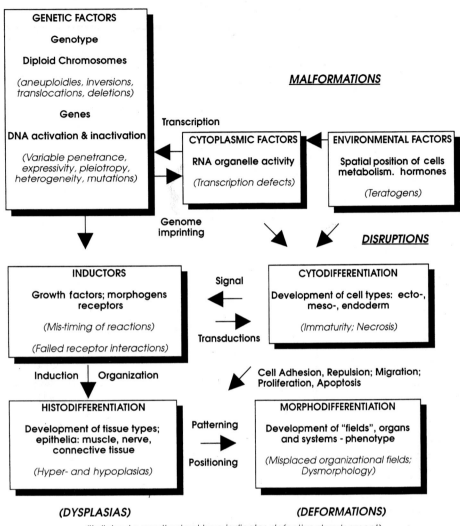

Figure 2–1 Schema of embryogenesis and possible sources of anomalies. (Defective developments are italicized.) (DNA = deoxyribonucleic acid; RNA = ribonucleic acid)

The expressed character of differentiated cells (the phenotype) will depend on (1) their genetic constitution (the genotype) and (2) the type and degree of gene expression and repression and of environmental influences during differentiation. Defective genes (mutations) or abnormal chromosome numbers (aneuploidy or polyploidy) will pattern aberrant development. Adverse environmental factors, both prenatal and postnatal, can cause the genotypic pattern to deviate from normal development. Heredity (the genotype) and environment never work separately in patterning development but always work in combination to produce the phenotype.

Disturbances of the inductive patterns of embryonic tissues will result in congenital defects of development. Teratology constitutes the study of such abnormal development. Malformations of the face and jaws are frequently part of congenital abnormality syndromes that may be amenable to surgical, orthopedic, orthodontic, or therapeutic correction.

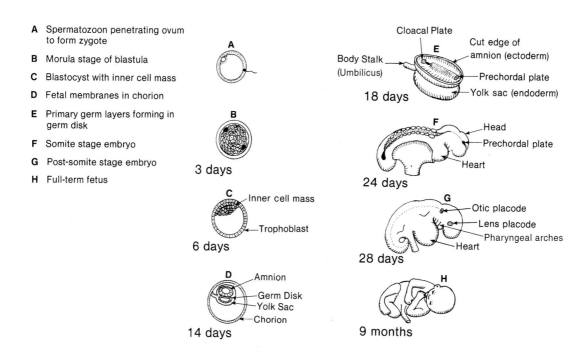

A Spermatozoon penetrating ovum to form zygote

B Morula stage of blastula

C Blastocyst with inner cell mass

D Fetal membranes in chorion

E Primary germ layers forming in germ disk

F Somite stage embryo

G Post-somite stage embryo

H Full-term fetus

Figure 2–2 Schematized synopsis of salient features of general embryology.

GROWTH

Growth is a fundamental attribute of developing organisms. The dramatic increase in size that characterizes the living embryo is a consequence of (1) the increased number of cells resulting from mitotic divisions (hyperplasia), (2) the increased size of individual cells (hypertrophy), and (3) the increased amount of noncellular material (accretion). Hyperplasia tends to predominate in the early embryo whereas hypertrophy largely prevails later. Once differentiation of a tissue has been established, further development is predominantly that of growth. The rate of tissue growth is inherently determined but is, of course, also dependent on environmental conditions. The health, diet, race, and sex of an individual influence the rate and extent of growth.

Growth may be interstitial, where an increase in bulk occurs within a tissue or organ, or appositional, where surface deposition of tissue enlarges its size. Interstitial growth characterizes soft tissues whereas hard tissues (bone, dental tissues) necessarily increase by apposition.

Growth is not merely an increase in size; if it were, the embryo would expand like a balloon, and the adult would simply be an enlarged fetus. The resulting unproportioned growth would produce a grossly distorted adult with a head as large as the rest of the body. Not all tissues, organs, and parts develop at the same rate, differential growth accounting for a varying proportional increase in size. The head is precocious in its development, constituting half the body size in the fetus but later undergoing a relative decrease in relation to total body size. Each organ system grows at its own predetermined

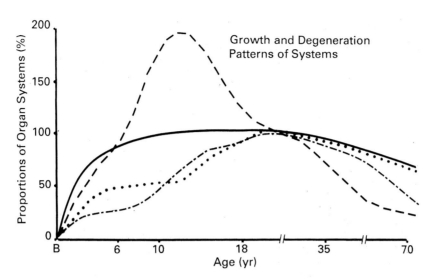

Figure 2–3 Graphic representation of the varying proportions of the various organ systems in postnatal life, where 100 percent represents the size of the organ systems in the mature young adult; ▬▬▬▬, lymphoid system;▬▬▬, central nervous system;▬·▬·▬, dentition;• • • • •, general body.) (Based on Scammon RE. The measurement of man. Minneapolis: University of Minnesota Press; 1930.)

rate, accounting for proportional discrepancies in size at different periods of life. Some organ systems enlarge precociously at first and subsequently remain nearly unchanged in size whereas others continue to grow until adolescence. For example, the lymphoid system (tonsils, thymus, etc.) continues to grow until adolescence. After extremely rapid growth in early childhood, the lymphoid system even regresses in size before adulthood (Fig. 2–3).

Incremental growth changes vary with chronologic age, being most rapid in the fetus and infant and rapid again at puberty. Despite the varying growth rates of different organ systems, there is an overall harmony of proportions. As an example, teeth are initiated and grow at the precise time at which the jaws are large enough to accommodate them.

The apparently scattered order of eruption of the teeth is another manifestation of the phenomenon of differing rates of growth. Teeth of various categories erupt at different times. The growth and development sequence is genetically determined and operates through the mechanism of inductors, metabolic modulators, neurotrophic and hormonal substances, and interacting systems of contact stimulation and inhibition of contiguous tissues. Should these differential but integrated rates of development fail to maintain their normal determined "pace," aberrations of overall development will manifest themselves as malformations that may require clinical correction.

Maturation is a counterpart of growth. Maturation indicates not only the attainment of adult size and proportions but also the attainment of the full adult constituents of tissues (eg, mineralization) as well as the complete capability of each organ to perform its destined functions.

When the age of occurrence of maturational events is indicated (onset of ossification centers, fusion of sutures, eruption of teeth, etc.), it must be stressed that these manifestations of the biologic age of an individual need not coincide with chronologic age, and in fact, the two ages often differ from one

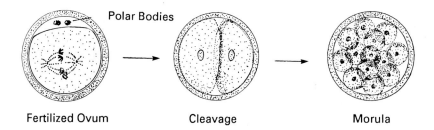

Polar Bodies

Fertilized Ovum   Cleavage   Morula

Figure 2–4 Initial stages of embryogenesis, depicting cell division. Note that the morula, containing up to 16 cells, is no larger than the fertilized ovum.

another. When biologic age is well in advance of chronologic age, the individual develops rapidly; when the reverse occurs, the individual has a retarded rate of development.

Although most growth normally ceases at the end of adolescence, coinciding with the eruption of the third molar teeth (hence the popular connotation of "wisdom" teeth), the facial bones, unlike the long bones, retain the potential for further appositional growth in adult life. Such postadolescent growth may occur as a result of hypersecretion of somatotrophic hormone from a pituitary gland tumor, as in acromegaly, which is characterized by enlargement of the bones of the face, hands, and feet.

PHASES OF DEVELOPMENT

Embryogenesis is divided into three distinct phases during the 280 days of gestation (composed of ten 28-day menstrual cycles):* the preimplantation period (the first 7 days), the embryonic period (the next 7 weeks), and the fetal period (the next 7 calendar months).

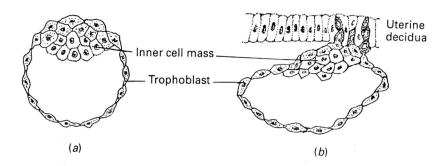

Inner cell mass

Trophoblast

Uterine decidua

(a)   (b)

Figure 2–5 The blastocyst (a), developed from the morula, implants (b) into the decidual layer of the uterine wall.

---

*This duration of gestation is based upon the menstrual cycle of 28 days. Calculation from the last occurring menstruation is known as the "menstrual age" of the embryo. As it is based upon the last occurrence of an easily observed event, menstrual age is most frequently used in obstetric practice. As ovulation and subsequent fertilization occur approximately 14 days after the last menstruation, the true age of the embryo ("fertilization age") is 2 weeks less than the menstrual age. Because fertilization age is more accurate, all ages referred to hereafter are fertilization ages unless otherwise specified. To distinguish from postnatal ages, prenatal ages are indicated as being post conception.

TABLE 2–1 Chronology of events during the embryonic period

Carnegie Stage	Postconception Age	Craniofacial Features
6	14 days	Primitive streak appears; oropharyngeal membrane forms
8	17 days	Neural plate forms
9	20 days	Cranial neural folds elevate; otic placode appears
10	21 days	Neural crest migration commences; fusion of neural folds; otic pit forms
11	24 days	Frontonasal prominence swells; first arch forms; wide stomodeum; optic vesicles form; anterior neuropore closes; olfactory placode appears
12	26 days	Second arch forms; maxillary prominences appear; lens placodes commence; posterior neuropore closes; adenohypophysial pouch appears
13	28 days	Third arch forms; dental lamina appears; fourth arch forms; oropharyngeal membrane ruptures
14	32 days	Otic and lens vesicles present; lateral nasal prominences appear
15	33 days	Medial nasal prominences appear; nasal pits form-widely separated, face laterally
16	37	Nasal pits face ventrally; upper lip forms on lateral aspect of stomodeum; lower lip fuses in midline; retinal pigment forms; nasolacrimal groove appears, demarcating nose; neurohypophysial evagination
17	41 days	Contact between medial nasal and maxillary prominences, separating nasal pit from stomodeum; upper lip continuity first established; vomeronasal organ appears
18	44 days	Primary palate anlagen project posteriorly into stomodeum; distinct tip of nose develops; eyelid folds form; retinal pigment; nasal pits move medially; nasal alae and septum present; mylohyoid, geniohyoid and genioglossus muscles form
19	47-48 days	Nasal fin disintegrates; (failure of disintegration predisposes to cleft lip); the rima oris of the mouth diminishes in width; mandibular ossification commences
20	50-51 days	The lidless eyes migrate medially; nasal pits approach each other; ear hillocks fuse
22	54 days	The eyelids thicken and encroach upon the eyes; the auricle forms and projects; the nostrils are in definitive position
23	56-57 days	Eyes are still wide apart but eyelid closure commences; nose tip elevates; face assumes a human fetal appearance; head elevates off the thorax; mouth opens; palatal shelves elevate; maxillary ossification commences
Fetus	60 days	Palatal shelves fuse; deciduous tooth buds form; embryo now termed a fetus

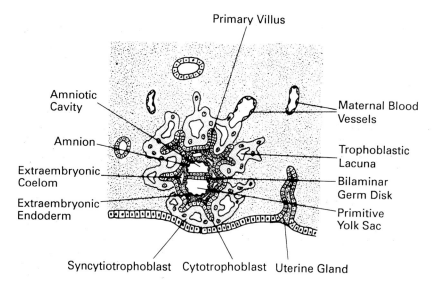

Figure 2–6 A 10-day-old conceptus implanted in the uterine wall. The fetal membranes, amnion, yolk sac, and chorion (syncytiotrophoblast and cytotrophoblast) have formed. The forming placenta surrounds the conceptus.

The Preimplantation Period

During the first 2 to 3 days post conception, the zygote progresses from a single cell to a 16-cell cluster, the morula, no larger than the original ovum (Fig. 2–4). The early totipotential blastomeres can develop into any tissue, but later differentiation creates an approximately 100-cell fluid-filled blastocyst. The outer sphere of cells forms the trophoblast, and the inner cell mass will form the embryo (Fig. 2–5). During this period, the conceptus passes along the uterine tube to enter the uterus, where it implants into the uterine endometrium on the 7th postconception day. The trophoblast converts into the chorion by sprouting villi. Chorionic implantation establishes the placenta, the organ of fetomaternal exchange of nutrition and waste disposal (Fig. 2–6).

The Embryonic Period

This phase, from the end of the 1st week until the 8th week, can be subdivided into three periods: presomite (8 to 21 days post conception), somite (21 to 31 days), and postsomite (32 to 56 days). During the presomite period, the primary germ layers of the embryo and the embryonic adnexa (fetal membranes) are formed in the inner cell mass. In the somite period, characterized by the appearance of prominent dorsal metameric segments, the basic patterns of the main body systems and organs are established. The postsomite period is characterized by the formation of the body's external features. The chronology of events occurring during the embryonic period, subdivided into stages, is designated in Table 2–1.

The Fetal Period

The beginning of this long phase (from the 8th week until term) is identified by the first appearance of ossification centers and by the earliest movements by the fetus. There is little new tissue differentiation or organogenesis, but there is rapid growth and expansion of the basic structures already formed.

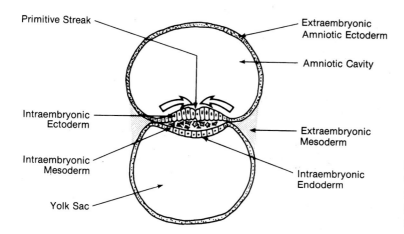

Figure 2–7 Cross-sectional view of the embryonic disk (center), fetal membranes amnion (above), and yolk sac (below).

THE FETAL MEMBRANES*

Embryonic adnexa form membranes surrounding cavities in which the embryo (and subsequently the fetus) develops. These fluid-filled cavities, membranes, and organs protect the fetus physically and serve its nutritional and waste disposal requirements, casting off at birth. The main cavities and their membranes are the chorion and amnion, surrounding the fetus. Lesser cavities and their membranes are the yolk sac and a transient diverticulum, the allantois, that become incorporated into the umbilical cord, connected to the placenta, the chief organ of fetal sustenance (Figs. 2–7 and 2–8; see also Fig. 2–6).

The chorion arises from the trophoblast as an all-encompassing membrane that along with the maternal endometrium forms the placenta. The amnion and yolk sac (fluid-filled sacs in the inner cell mass within the chorion) are separated by a bilaminar plate; this plate forms the embryonic disk, which later gives rise to the definitive embryo. The attachment of the inner cell mass to the

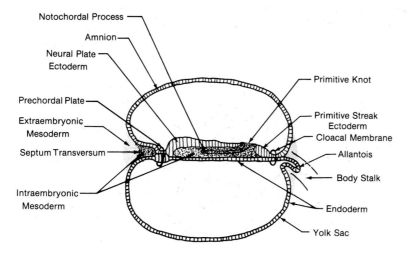

Figure 2–8 Longitudinal section through a 14-day-old embryo, depicting the fetal membranes (amnion, yolk sac, and allantois) and sites of ectoderm/endoderm contact (prechordal plate and cloacal membrane).

*The long-established term "fetal membranes" is a misnomer for the various extraembryonic structures collectively described under this title as these structures are not necessarily fetal or membranes. However, there is no suitable alternative nomenclature.

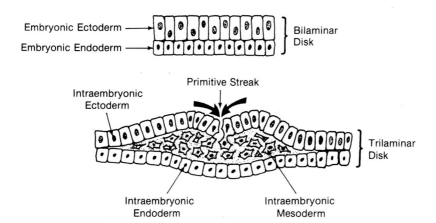

Figure 2–9
Schematic cross section of the embryonic disk at bilaminar (above) and trilaminar (below) stages. Enlarged view of the center of Fig. 2–7.

chorion constitutes the connecting (body) stalk that contains the yolk sac and allantois. The stalk converts into the umbilical cord.

EARLY EMBRYOGENESIS (EMBRYONIC PERIOD)

The Presomite Period

Development of Endoderm and Ectoderm

The primordial embryonic germ disk is composed of two primary germ layers: the ectoderm, which forms the floor of the amniotic cavity, and the endoderm, which forms the roof of the yolk sac (Fig. 2–9; also see Fig. 2–7). At the 14th day, there is early demarcation of the anterior pole of the initially oval disk: an endodermal thickening, the prechordal plate, appears in the future midcephalic region (Fig. 2–10). The prechordal plate is believed to perform a head-organizing function. Defects in the prechordal plate may result in holo-prosencephaly or agenesis of the corpus callosum. The prechordal plate gives rise to cephalic mesenchyme concerned with extrinsic eye muscle development. The prechordal plate also gives rise to the preoral gut (Seessel's pouch). The prechordal plate prefaces the development of the orofacial region, giving rise later to the endodermal layer of the oropharyngeal membrane; the importance of this membrane is discussed later in relation to development of the

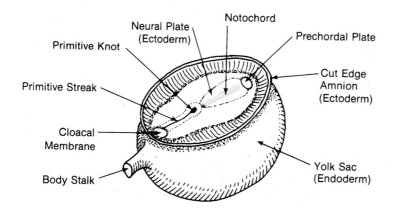

Figure 2–10 Dorsal surface view of the embryonic disk with the amnion cover removed. The prechordal plate demarcates the future mouth. The body stalk will form the umbilical cord connecting the embryo to the placenta.

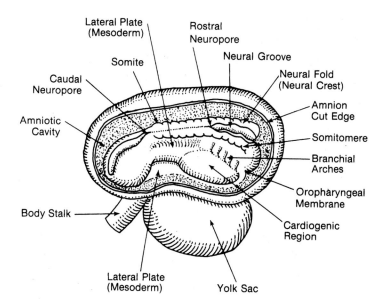

Figure 2–11 Lateral view of a 23-day-old embryo, depicting the fusion of neural folds. The somites are forming.

mouth. The third primary germ layer, the mesoderm, makes its appearance at the beginning of the 3rd week as a result of ectodermal cell proliferation and differentiation in the caudal region of the embryonic disk. The resultant bulge in the disk is grooved craniocaudally, for which it is termed the "primitive streak" (see Fig. 2–9). From the primitive streak, the rapidly proliferating tissue known as mesenchyme forms the intraembryonic mesoderm, which migrates in all directions between the ectoderm and endoderm except at the sites of the oropharyngeal membrane anteriorly and the cloacal membrane posteriorly (see Figs. 2–8 and 2–10). The appearance of the mesoderm converts the bilaminar disk into a trilaminar structure. The midline axis becomes defined by the formation of the notochord from the proliferation and differentiation of the cranial end of the primitive streak. The notochord serves as the axial skeleton of the embryo and induces formation of the neural plate in the overlying ectoderm (neural ectoderm). The lateral mesoderm induces epidermal development (cutaneous ectoderm) (Figs. 2–11 and 2–12).

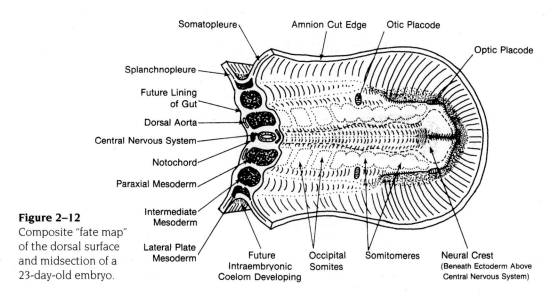

Figure 2–12 Composite "fate map" of the dorsal surface and midsection of a 23-day-old embryo.

TABLE 2–2 Derivatives of Neural Crest Cells

Connective tissues

Ectomesenchyme of facial prominences and pharyngeal arches
Bones and cartilages of facial and visceral skeleton (basicranial and pharyngeal-arch cartilages)
Dermis of face and ventral aspect of neck
Stroma of salivary, thymus, thyroid, parathyroid, and pituitary glands
Corneal mesenchyme
Sclera and choroid optic coats
Blood-vessel walls (excepting endothelium); aortic arch arteries
Dental papilla (dentine); portion of periodontal ligament; cementum

Muscle tissues

Ciliary muscles
Covering connective tissues of pharyngeal-arch muscles (masticatory, facial, faucial, laryngeal)
  combined with mesodermal components

Nervous tissues

Supporting tissues
  Leptomeninges of prosencephalon and part of mesencephalon
  Glia
  Schwann's sheath cells
Sensory ganglia
  Autonomic ganglia
  Spinal dorsal root ganglia
  Sensory ganglia (in part) of trigeminal, facial (geniculate), glossopharyngeal (otic and superior),
    and vagal (jugular) nerves
Autonomic nervous system
  Sympathetic ganglia and plexuses
  Parasympathetic ganglia (ciliary, ethmoid, sphenopalatine, submandibular, and enteric system)

Endocrine tissues

Adrenomedullary cells and adrenergic paraganglia
Calcitonin parafollicular cells— thyroid gland (ultimopharyngeal body)
Carotid body

Pigment cells

Melanocytes in all tissues
Melanophores of iris

The three primary germ layers serve as a basis for differentiating the tissues and organs that are largely derived from each of the layers (see flowchart in Appendix, pg 206). The cutaneous and neural systems develop from the ectoderm. The cutaneous structures include the skin and its appendages, the oral

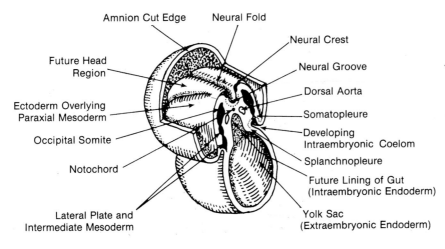

Amnion Cut Edge   Neural Fold
Neural Crest
Future Head Region
Neural Groove
Ectoderm Overlying Paraxial Mesoderm
Dorsal Aorta
Occipital Somite
Somatopleure
Developing Intraembryonic Coelom
Notochord
Splanchnopleure
Future Lining of Gut (Intraembryonic Endoderm)
Lateral Plate and Intermediate Mesoderm
Yolk Sac (Extraembryonic Endoderm)

Figure 2–13
Transverse section through a 20-day-old embryo, depicting neural folds and neural crest formation.

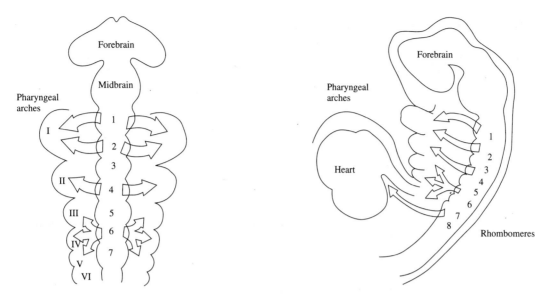

Figure 2–14 Schematic depiction of neural crest migration pathways from rhombomeres 1 to 7 to pharyngeal arches labeled I to VI, from dorsal (left) and lateral (right) aspects. (From Ann Acad Singapore 1999;28: 708–13)

mucous membrane, and the enamel of teeth. The neural structures include the central and peripheral nervous systems. The mesoderm gives rise to the cardiovascular system (heart and blood vessels), the locomotor system (bones and muscles), connective tissues, and dental pulp. The endoderm develops into the lining epithelium of the respiratory system and of the alimentary canal between the pharynx and the anus, as well as the secretory cells of the liver and pancreas.

Development of the ectoderm into its cutaneous and neural portions, by fibroblast growth factor (FGF) signaling, occurs at 20 to 22 days by the infolding of the neural plate ectoderm along the midline forming the neural folds; this creates a neural groove in the process of neurulation. At 22 days, the neural folds fuse in the region of the third to fifth somites, the site of the future nuchal

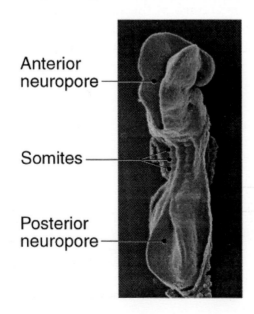

Figure 2–15 Scanning electron micrograph of a mouse embryo equivalent to a 22-day-old human embryo with 4 to 12 pairs of somites. The neural folds have fused in the future hindbrain region. (Courtesy of Dr. K. K. Sulik)

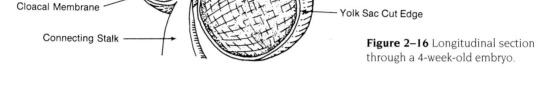

Figure 2–16 Longitudinal section through a 4-week-old embryo.

region. Further multiple initial closure sites proceed both cephalically and caudally to form the neural tube, which submerges beneath the superficial covering of the cutaneous ectoderm (Fig. 2–13; also see Figs. 2–11 and 2–20). The lens and otic placodes, which will form the eye lenses and inner ears, appear on the surface ectoderm at this stage. The anterior and posterior neuropores close at 25 and 27 days, respectively.

Development of the Neural Crest

This ectomesenchymal tissue, termed the neural crest from its site of origin (see Fig. 2–13), arises from the crests of the neural folds where neuralizing and epidermalizing influences interact. Neural crest cells form a separate tissue that, being akin to the three primary germ layers, is pluripotential. Neural crest ectomesenchyme possesses great migratory propensities, following natural cleavage planes between mesoderm, ectoderm, and endoderm and tracking intramesodermally. These population shifts may be either passive

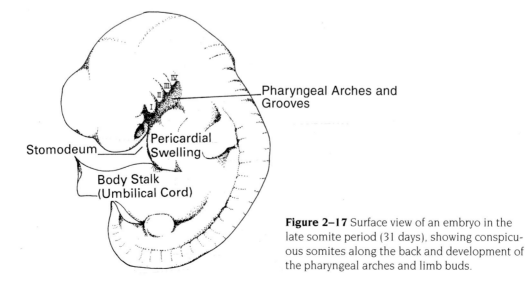

Figure 2–17 Surface view of an embryo in the late somite period (31 days), showing conspicuous somites along the back and development of the pharyngeal arches and limb buds.

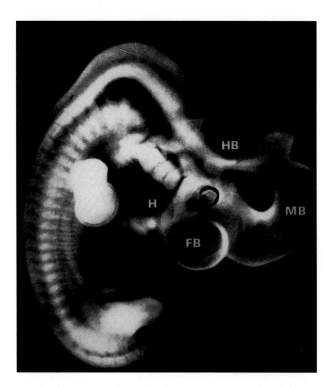

Figure 2–18 Lateral view of a human embryo in the late somite period (early in the 5th week). Note the forebrain (FB), containing the prominent eye, and the midbrain (MB) and hindbrain (HB). The primitive face is flexed in contact with the prominent heart (H). The somites are evident as dorsal segments continuing into a tail. The upper and lower limb buds are seen as prominent paddle-shaped projections. (Courtesy of the late Professor Dr. E. Blechschmidt)

translocations (resulting from displacement of tissues) or active cell migrations. Translocated neural crest cells, upon reaching their predetermined destinations, undergo cytodifferentiation into a wide variety of diverse cell types that are in part genetically predetermined and in part specified by local environmental influences (Table 2–2). Neural crest cells divide as they migrate, forming a larger population at their destination than at their origin. These cells form the major source of connective-tissue components, including cartilage, bone, and ligaments of the facial and oral regions, and contribute to the muscles and arteries of these regions.

Cranial neural crest tissue is discontinuous and segments into regions adjacent to the brain. Neural crest cell clusters adjacent to the neural tube form the ganglia of the autonomic nervous system and sensory nerves. Neural crest from the hindbrain arises from segments known as rhombomeres. Crest tissue from rhombomeres 1 and 2 migrates into the first pharyngeal arch; neural crest from rhombomere 4 migrates into the second arch, and from rhombomeres 6 and 7, into the third, fourth, and sixth arches. Rhombomeres 3 and 5 are free of neural crest (Fig. 2–14).

The neural crest cells, being multipotential, display varying regional characteristics at their destination sites. Those remaining rostral and dorsal to the forebrain contribute to the leptomeninges and parts of the skull. Those around the midbrain form part of the anlage of the trigeminal nerve ganglion; in conjunction with the cranial paraxial mesoderm, they form the chondrocranium (see

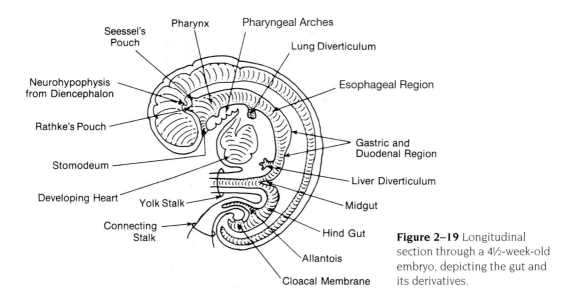

Seessel's Pouch

Pharynx

Pharyngeal Arches

Lung Diverticulum

Neurohypophysis from Diencephalon

Esophageal Region

Rathke's Pouch

Gastric and Duodenal Region

Stomodeum

Liver Diverticulum

Developing Heart

Yolk Stalk

Midgut

Connecting Stalk

Hind Gut

Allantois

Cloacal Membrane

Figure 2–19 Longitudinal section through a 4½-week-old embryo, depicting the gut and its derivatives.

Chapter 8). Interaction with an epithelium (neural or epidermal) is necessary before chondrogenesis can begin.

Neural crest cells migrating ventrally and caudally encounter the pharyngeal endoderm that induces formation of the pharyngeal arches. Many pharyngeal derivatives, including facial bones, are of neural crest origin (see Chapter 4). Those cells that migrate within cranial paraxial mesoderm form somitomeres, which provide most of the muscles of the face and jaws. Other neural crest cells provide mesenchyme for angiogenesis to produce blood vessels; yet others are the source of melanocytes for skin and eye pigmentation.

The developing craniofacial complex is a community of all the above cell populations. Deviation of any one of these populations from its normal development and spatial cueing has deleterious consequences, inducing clusters of anomalies termed neurocristopathy syndromes.

The Somite Period

The basic tissue types having developed during the first 21 days, development is characterized during the next 10 days by foldings and structuring as well as by differentiation of the basic tissues that convert the flat embryonic disk into a tubular body (Figs. 2–15 and 2–16; also see Figs. 2–11, 2–12, and 2–14). The first of these changes (21 days) is the folding of the neural plate, from which the brain and spinal cord develop. Next, the mesoderm develops into three aggregations—the lateral plate, intermediate, and paraxial mesoderm, each with a different fate. The lateral plate mesoderm contributes to the walls of the embryonic coelom from which the pleural, pericardial, and peritoneal cavities develop. Lateral mesoderm also forms peripharyngeal connective tissues of the neck. The intermediate mesoderm, absent from the head region, contributes to the formation of the gonads, kidneys, and adrenal cortex. The paraxial mesoderm, alongside the notochord, forms a rostral condensation of incompletely segmented somitomeres. The cranial somitomeric mesoderm migrates into the ventral pharyngeal region to contribute to the future pharyngeal arches (Fig. 2–17). The caudal paraxial mesoderm forms a series of segmental blocks, termed somites; their prominence characterizes this period (days 21 to 31) of embryonic development (Fig. 2–18; also see Fig. 2–17). The 42 to 44 paired somites appear sequentially craniocaudally and set the pattern for the regions of the body by their being identified as 4 occipital, 8 cervical, 12 thoracic, 5 lumbar, 5 sacral, and 8 to 10 coccygeal somites (see Figs. 2–17 and 2–18).

Each somite differentiates into three parts; their fates are implied by their names. The ventromedial part is designated the sclerotome;* it contributes to the vertebral column and accounts for its segmental nature, except in the occipital region, where fusion forms the occipital skull bone. The lateral aspect of the somite, termed the dermatome, gives rise to the dermis of the skin. The intermediate portion, the myotome, differentiates into muscles of the trunk and limbs and contributes to some of the muscles of the orofacial region.

The somite period is characterized by the establishment of most of the organ systems of the embryo. The cardiovascular, alimentary, respiratory, genitourinary, and nervous systems are established, and the primordia of the eye and the internal ear appear. The embryonic disk develops lateral, head, and tail folds, facilitating enclosure of the endodermal germ layer from the yolk sac, thereby laying the basis for the tubular intestine. The part of the yolk sac endoderm incorporated into the cranial end of the embryo is termed the foregut, the anterior boundary of which is closed off by the oropharyngeal membrane. Similarly, the part of the yolk sac incorporated into the caudal end of the embryo is termed the hindgut, and is bounded ventrally by the cloacal membrane. The intervening portion of the alimentary canal is called the midgut; this remains in communication with the yolk sac through the yolk stalk (Fig. 2–19). The gut is initially sealed off at both ends and is converted into a canal only by the later breakdown of the oropharyngeal and cloacal membranes.

The foregut endoderm later gives rise to the laryngotracheal diverticulum, from which the bronchi and lungs develop. Other endodermal outgrowths from the foregut are the hepatic and pancreatic diverticula, which give rise to the secretory elements of the liver and pancreas. The foregut itself develops into the pharynx and its important pharyngeal pouches, the esophagus, the stomach, and the first part of the duodenum. The midgut forms the rest of the duodenum, the entire small intestine, and the ascending and transverse colon of the large intestine. The hindgut forms the descending colon and the terminal parts of the alimentary canal.

The external appearance of the late somite embryo presents a prominent brain forming a predominant portion of the early head, whose "face" and "neck," formed by pharyngeal arches, are strongly flexed over a precocious heart. The eyes, nose, and ears are demarcated by placodes while ventrolateral swellings indicate the beginnings of the limb buds. The lower belly wall protrudes conspicuously in its connections with the placenta through the connecting (body) stalk, and a prominent tail terminates the caudal end of the embryo (see Figs. 2–17 and 2–18).

---

*Proteoglycans (procollagen) and collagen secreted by the notochord induce the conversion of somite sclerotomal cells into cartilage.

The extremely complex and rapid basic organogenesis taking place during the 10-day somite period makes the embryo exceedingly susceptible to environmental disturbances that may produce permanent developmental derangements. Maternal illnesses, particularly of viral origin, and irradiation and drug therapy during the first trimester of pregnancy (which includes the somite period of development) are well known in obstetric practice to be the cause of some congenital anomalies of the fetus.

The Postsomite Period

The predominance of the segmental somites as an external feature of the early embryo fades during the 6th week post conception. The head dominates much of the development of this period. Facial features become recognizable as the ears, eyes, and nose assume a "human" form and as the neck becomes defined by its elongation and by the sheathing of the pharyngeal arches. The paddle-shaped limb buds of the early part of the period expand and differentiate into their divisions to the first demarcation of their digits. The earliest muscular movements are first manifest at this time. The body stalk of the previous periods condenses into a definitive umbilical cord as it becomes less conspicuous on the belly wall. The thoracic region swells enormously as the heart, which becomes very prominent in the somite period, is joined by the rapidly growing liver, whose size dominates the early abdominal organs. The long tail of the beginning of the embryonic period regresses as the growing buttocks aid in its concealment. The embryo at the end of this period is now termed a fetus.

The Fetal Period

The main organs and systems having developed during the embryonic period, the last 7 months of fetal life are devoted to very rapid growth and reproportioning of body components, with little further organogenesis or tissue differentiation. The precocious growth and development of the head in the embryonic period is not maintained in the fetal period, with the result that the body develops relatively more rapidly. The proportions of the head are thereby reduced from about half the overall body length at the beginning of the fetal period to about one-third at the 5th month and to about one-fourth at birth. At 4 months post conception, the face assumes a human appearance as the laterally directed eyes move to the front of the face and as the ears rise to eye level from their original mandibulocervical site. The limbs grow rapidly but disproportionately, the lower limbs more slowly than the upper. Ossification centers make their appearance in most of the bones during this period. The sex of the fetus can be observed externally by the 3rd month, and the wrinkled skin acquires a covering of downy hairs (lanugo) by the 5th month. During this month, fetal movements are first felt by the mother. The sebaceous glands of the skin become very active just before birth (7th and 8th months), covering the fetus with their fatty secretions, termed the vernix caseosa (*vernix*, varnish; *caseosa*, cheesy). Fat makes its first appearance in the face when adipose tissue differentiates and proliferates from the 14th week post conception onwards. It appears initially in the buccal fat pad area, then in the cheek, and finally in the chin subcutis. In the last 2 months of fetal life, fat is deposited subcutaneously to fill out the wrinkled skin, and nearly half the ultimate birth weight is added.

Despite the rapid growth of the postcranial portions of the body during the fetal period, the head still has the largest circumference of all the parts of the body at birth. The passage of the head through the birth canal is accommodated by its compression. The compression of the cranium at birth presents the danger of distortion; this compression normally rectifies itself postnatally, but it may persist as a source of perverted mandibulofacial development.

ANOMALIES OF DEVELOPMENT

Neural tube defects leading to a spectrum of congenital anomalies varying from mere disfigurement to lethal conditions are among the more common congenital anomalies. Such defects are attributed to (among other causes) deficiencies of nutritional folic acid, a water-soluble vitamin. Adequate folic acid intake during early pregnancy minimizes the incidence of neural tube defects.

Neural tube closure occurs at several sites, as shown in Fig. 2–20. Closure is initiated at the boundary between the future hindbrain and the spinal cord (site 1) and at three distinct sites in the cranial region (sites 2, 3, and 4). A fifth closure site, involving a process of canalization, occurs in the caudal region (site 5). The directions of closure are indicated by the arrows. Failure of closure results in neural tube defects, as shown in the right hand panels of Fig. 2–20. The top row depicts anencephaly and craniorachischisis. Encephaloceles (middle row)

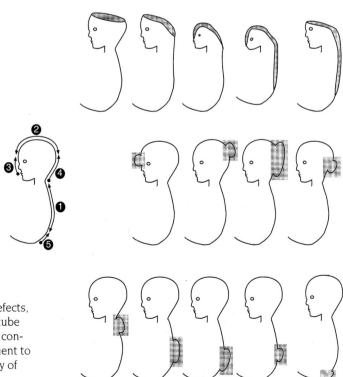

Figure 2–20 Schematic depiction of neural tube defects, sites of sequential neural-tube closure points (1 to 5) and congenital anomalies consequent to failure of closure. (Courtesy of Dr. D. Alan Underhill)

involve failures to complete neural tube closure or membrane fusion at closure points (sites 2, 3, and 4) within the cranial region. Spina bifida cystica (bottom row) comprises a range of neural tube defects of the spinal cord and its coverings at various levels (sites 1 and 5).

Selected Bibliography

Anderson DJ. Cellular and molecular biology of neural crest cell lineage determination. Trends Genet 1997;13:276–80.

Anthony AC, Hansen DK. Hypothesis: folate-responsive neural tube defects and neurocristopathies. Teratology 2000;62:42–50.

Garcia-Castro M, Bronner-Fraser M. Induction and differentiation of the neural crest. Curr Opin Cell Biol 1999;11:695–8.

Johnson MC, Bronsky PT. Embryonic craniofacial development. Prog Clin Biol Res 1991;373:99–115.

Johnson MC, Bronsky PT. Prenatal craniofacial development: new insights on normal and abnormal mechanisms. Crit Rev Oral Biol Med 1995;6:368–422.

Kanzler B, Foreman RK, Labosky PA, Mallo M. BMP signaling is essential for development of skeletogenic and neurogenic cranial neural crest. Development 2000;127:1095–1104.

Kjaer I. Human prenatal craniofacial development related to brain development under normal and pathologic conditions. Acta Odontol Scand 1995;53:135–43.

La Bonne C, Bronner-Fraser M. Molecular mechanisms of neural crest formation. Annu Rev Cell Dev Biol 1999;15:81–112.

Lallier TE. Cell lineage and cell migration in the neural crest. Ann N Y Acad Sci 1991;615:158–71.

Nakatsu T, Uwabe C, Shiota K. Neural tube closure in humans initiates at multiple sites: evidence from human embryos and implications for the pathogenesis of neural tube defects. Anat Embryol 2000;201:455–66.

O'Rahilly R, Müller F. Minireview: summary of the initial development of the human nervous system. Teratology 1999;60:39–41.

O'Rahilly R, Müller F. Prenatal ages and stages—measures and errors. Teratology 2000;61:382–4.

O'Rahilly R, Müller F. The embryonic human brain. 2nd ed. New York: Wiley-Liss; 1999.

Perris R, Perissinotto D. Role of the extracellular matrix during neural crest cell migration. Mech Dev 2000;95:3–21.

Streit A, Berliner AJ, Papanayotou C, et al. Initiation of neural induction by FGF signalling before gastrulation. Nature 2000;406:74–8.

Tanaka O. Variabilities in prenatal development of orofacial system. Anat Anz 1991;172:97–107.

Web Sites

Embryo images [accessed 2000 July 27].
URL:http://www.med.unc.edu/embryo_images/

3 EARLY OROFACIAL DEVELOPMENT

Development of the head depends on the inductive activities of the prosencephalic and rhombencephalic organizing centers, which are regulated by the sonic hedgehog (SHH) gene that is expressed as a signaling protein in the notochord and the neural floor plate cells (Fig. 3–1). The prosencephalic center, derived from prechordal mesoderm that migrates from the primitive streak, is at the rostral end of the notochord beneath the forebrain (prosencephalon); it induces the visual and inner-ear apparatus and upper third of the face. The caudal rhombencephalic center induces the middle and lower thirds of the face (the viscerofacial skeleton), including the middle and external ears.

Associated with these developments is the division of the initially unilobar forebrain (Fig. 3–2) into paired telencephalic hemispheres and evagination of the paired olfactory bulbs and optic nerves. Failure of these cerebral divisions (holoprosencephaly) has a profound influence on facial development, leading to many types of anomalies.

Oral development in the embryo is demarcated extremely early in life by the appearance of the prechordal plate in the bilaminar germ disk on the 14th day of development, even before the mesodermal germ layer appears. The endodermal thickening of the prechordal plate designates the cranial pole of the oval embryonic disk and later contributes to the oropharyngeal membrane. This tenuous and temporary bilaminar membrane is the site of the junction of the ectoderm that forms the mucosa of the mouth and the endoderm that forms the mucosa of the pharynx, which is the most cranial part of the foregut. The oropharyngeal membrane is one of two sites of contiguity between ectoderm and endoderm, where mesoderm fails to intervene between the two primary germ layers; the other site is the cloacal membrane at the terminal end of the hindgut. The oropharyngeal membrane also demarcates the site of a shallow depression (the stomodeum), the primitive mouth that forms the topographic center of the developing face.

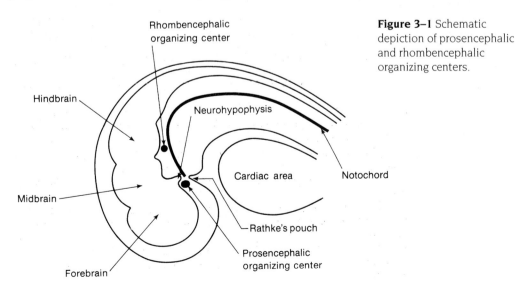

Figure 3–1 Schematic depiction of prosencephalic and rhombencephalic organizing centers.

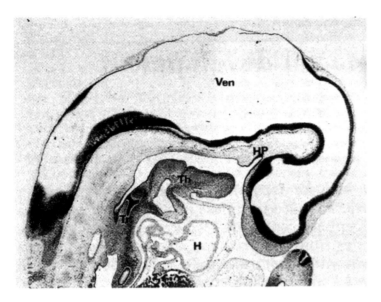

Figure 3–2 Sagittal section of the head region of a 32-day-old embryo. The ventricles (Ven) occupy a large proportion of the brain. The hypophysial pouch (HP) extends up from the stomodeum, which is bordered below by the heart (H). The thyroid gland (Th) is budding from the foramen caecum in the tongue via the thyroglossal duct. The trachea (Tr) is budding from the primitive esophagus. (×22 original magnification) (Courtesy of Professor H. Nishimura).

Rapid orofacial development is characteristic of the more advanced development of the cranial portion of the embryo over that of its caudal portion. The differential rates of growth result in a pear-shaped embryonic disk, the head region forming the expanded portion of the pear (see Fig. 2–10 in Chapter 2).

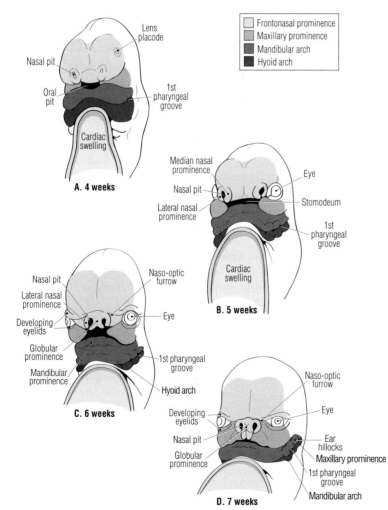

Figure 3–3 Schematic depiction of facial formation at 4, 5, 6, and 7 weeks post conception.

Further, the three germ layers in the cranial part of the embryo begin their specific development by the middle of the 3rd week whereas separation of the germ layers continues in the caudal portion until the end of the 4th week. Because of the precocious development of the cranial end of the embryo, the head constitutes nearly half the total body size during the postsomite embryonic period (5th to 8th weeks); with subsequent postcranial development, it forms only one-quarter of the body length at birth but 6 to 8 percent of the body in adulthood.

FORMATION OF THE FACE

The face derives from five prominences that surround a central depression, the stomodeum, which constitutes the future mouth. The prominences are the single median frontonasal and the paired maxillary and mandibular prominences (Figs. 3–3 and 3–4); the latter two are derivatives of the first pair of six pharyngeal arches. All of these prominences and arches arise from neural crest ectomesenchyme that migrates from its initial dorsal location into the facial and neck regions.

The frontonasal prominence surrounds the forebrain, which sprouts lateral optic diverticula that form the eyes. The frontal portion of the prominence between the eyes forms the forehead; at the inferolateral corners, thickened ectodermal nasal (olfactory) placodes arise (Fig. 3–5). These placodes become the olfactory epithelium and develop the underlying olfactory nerves. The placodes invaginate by the elevation of inverted horseshoe-shaped ridges, the

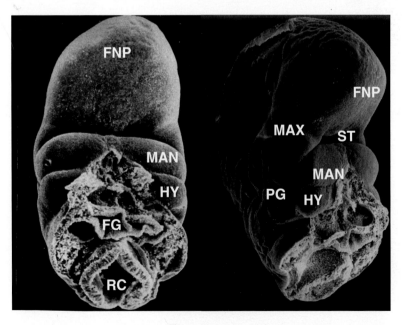

Figure 3–4 Scanning electron micrographs of the head region of a 26-day-old human embryo. The central stomodeum (ST) is bordered by the frontonasal prominence (FNP) above, the maxillary (MAX) prominences laterally, and the mandibular (MAN) prominences inferiorly. The hyoid (HY) arch borders the first pharyngeal groove (PG). The sectioned surface reveals the foregut (FG) and the rhombencephalon (RC). (Scale bar = 0.1 mm) (Reproduced with permission from Hinrichsen K. The early development of morphology and patterns of the face in the human embryo. In: Advances in anatomy, embryology and cell biology, 98, Springer-Verlag; 1985.)

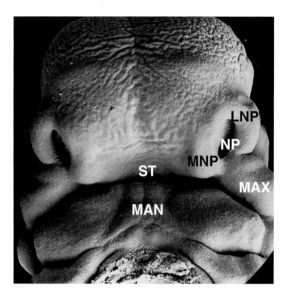

Figure 3–5 Scanning electron micrograph of the face of a 37-day-old human embryo. The nasal pits (NP) are surrounded by the medial (MNP) and lateral (LNP) nasal prominences and the maxillary (MAX) prominences. The wide stomodeum (ST) is limited inferiorly by the mandibular prominence (MAN). (Reproduced with permission from Hinrichson K. The early development of morphology and patterns of the face in the human embryo. In: Advances in anatomy, embryology and cell biology, 98. Springer-Verlag; 1985.)

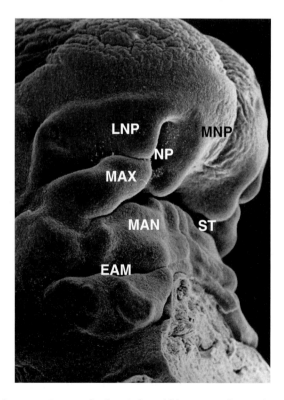

Figure 3–6 Scanning electron micrograph of a 41-day-old human embryo. The maxillary prominence (MAX) is wedged between the lateral (LNP) and medial (MNP) nasal prominences surrounding the nasal pit (NP). The stomodeum (ST) is bordered inferiorly by the mandibular (MAN) prominence. Auricular hillocks are forming around the external acoustic meatus (EAM). (Scale bar = 0.1 mm) (Reproduced with permission from Hinrichson K. The early development of morphology and patterns of the face in the human embryo. In: Advances in anatomy, embryology and cell biology, 98. Springer-Verlag; 1985.)

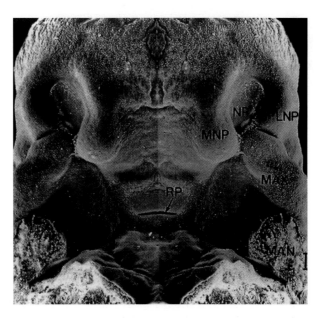

Figure 3–7 Scanning electron micrograph of the stomodeal chamber of a 41-day-old human embryo. The maxillary prominences (MAX) are wedged between the lateral (LNP) and medial (MNP) nasal prominences surrounding the nasal pits (NP). The mandibular prominences (MAN) are cut. Rathke's pouch (RP) is in the roof of the stomodeum. (Scale bar = 0.1 mm) (×65 original magnification) (Reproduced with permission from Hinrichson K. The early development of morphology and patterns of the face in the human embryo. In: Advances in anatomy, embryology and cell biology, 98. Springer-Verlag; 1985.)

medial and lateral nasal prominences, that surround each sinking nasal pit (Figs. 3–6 and 3–7). These pits are precursors of the anterior nares; the pits are initially in continuity with the stomodeum.

Union of the facial prominences occurs by either of two developmental events at different locations: merging of the frontonasal, maxillary, and mandibular prominences or fusion of the central maxillonasal components. Merging of what are initially incompletely separated prominences occurs as the intervening grooves disappear as a result of migration into and/or proliferation of underlying mesenchyme in the groove. Fusion of the freely projecting medial nasal prominences with the maxillary and lateral nasal prominences on each side requires the disintegration of their contacting surface epithelia (the nasal fin), allowing the underlying mesenchymal cells to intermingle. Failure of normal disintegration of the nasal fin by cell death or mesenchymal transformation is a cause of cleft upper lip and anterior palate, as such failure prevents the intermingling of maxillary and medial nasal mesenchyme.

Fusion of the medial nasal and maxillary prominences provides for continuity of the upper jaw and lip and separation of the nasal pits from the stomodeum. The midline merging of the medial nasal prominences forms the median tuberculum and philtrum of the upper lip, the tip of the nose, and the primary palate. The intermaxillary segment of the upper jaw (the premaxilla), in which the four upper incisor teeth will develop, arises from the median primary palate that is initially a widely separated pair of inwardly projecting swellings of the merged medial nasal prominences (see Fig. 3–7). Abnormal unilateral clefting resulting from failed fusion of medial nasal and maxillary

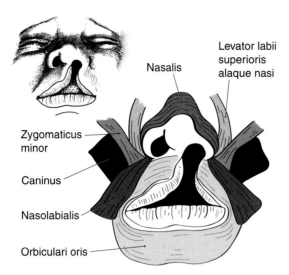

Figure 3–8 Schematic depiction of muscle orientation in unilateral cleft lip.

prominences produces a deflection of the nose and upper lip (globular process) (Fig. 3–8).

The lower jaw and lip are very simply formed by midline merging of the paired mandibular prominences and are the first parts of the face to become

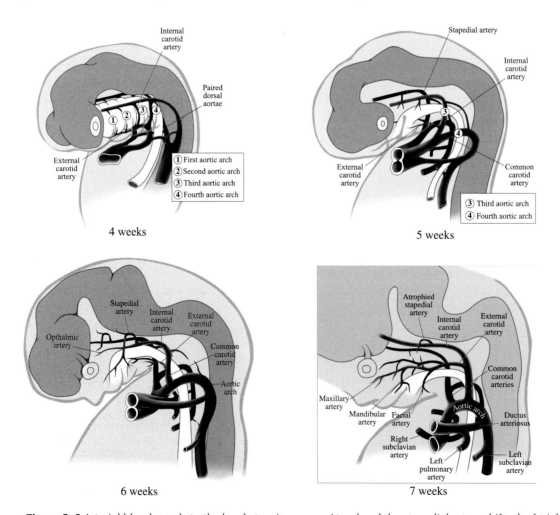

Figure 3–9 Arterial blood supply to the head at various ages. Atrophy of the stapedial artery shifts the facial blood supply from the internal to the external carotid artery.

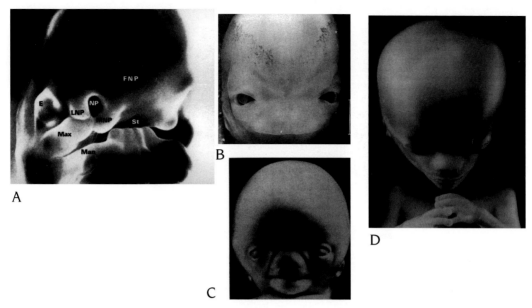

Figure 3–10 (*a*) Face of a human embryo in a late somite period (30 to 32 days). The frontonasal prominence (FNP) projects the medial nasal (MNP) and lateral nasal (LNP) prominences on each side, surrounding the nasal placode. The eye (E) is seen in its lateral position. The maxillary prominence (Max) forms the superolateral boundary of the stomodeum (St), and the mandibular prominence (Man) forms the lower boundary. (*b*) Photomicrograph of a 54-day-old human embryo, depicting widely separated eyes prior to eyelid closure. Note the superficial blood vessels in the forehead (scale bar = 1 mm). (*c*) Face of a 7-week-old human embryo. The relatively large forehead dominates the face. Eyelids are beginning to form above and below the migrating eyes. The mouth opening is becoming smaller. (*d*) Face of a 3-month-old fetus. The eyelids, their formation complete, are closed over the eyes. Medial migration of the eyes will narrow the interocular distance. Precocious brain development dominates the size of the head at this age. Ossification has started to form the craniofacial skeleton. (a, c and d courtesy of Prof. Dr. E. Blechschmidt; b reproduced with permission from Hinrichson K. The early development of morphology and patterns of the face in the human embryo. In: Advances in anatomy, embryology and cell biology, 98. Springer-Verlag; 1985.)

definitively established. The lateral merging of the maxillary and mandibular prominences creates the commissures (corners) of the mouth.

During the 7th week post conception, a shift in the blood supply of the face (from the internal to the external carotid artery) occurs as a result of normal atrophy of the stapedial artery (Fig. 3–9). This shift occurs at a critical time of midface and palate development, providing the potential for deficient blood supply and consequent defects of the upper lip and palate.

Not all regions of the face grow at the same rate during early development. There is a relative constancy of the central facial region (between the eyes) in relation to the rapidly expanding overall facial width. From 5 to 9 weeks, there is an actual reduction of interocular distance but an enlargement and consolidation of the other primordia, changes that confer human characteristics upon the developing face (Fig. 3–10, a to d). Malproportioning of growth during this time is the basis of developing craniofacial defects.

The Eyes

A median single field of cells—the optic primordium—in the anterior neural plate forming the ventral anterior diencephalon will develop bilateral retinas under the direction of the "cyclops" gene. Cyclopic signaling induces divergent morphogenetic movements of the ventral diencephalon to form bilateral eyes. The prechordal plate suppresses the median part of the optic

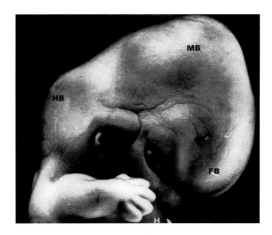

Figure 3–11 Lateral view of a 6½-week-old embryo. The face is strongly flexed over the prominent heart (H). Note the location of the forebrain (FB), midbrain (MB) and hindbrain (HB), and the first pharyngeal groove forming the external acoustic meatus. The fingers are differentiating out of the hand paddle Note the absence of eyelids and the prominent lens vesicle in the center of the optic cup. (Courtesy of the late Prof. Dr. E. Blechschmidt).

primordium to form bilateral primordia. The ventral anterior diencephalon fails to form in the absence or mutation of the cyclops gene, resulting in a single cyclopic eye.

Lateral expansions of initial forebrain evaginations (optic sulci) form optic vesicles, which medially retain their diencephalic (forebrain) connections (the optic stalks) and laterally induce thickened epithelial lens placodes on the sides of the future face (see Fig. 3–10, a). Invagination of the lens placode concomitantly with formation of optic vesicles creates the deep-set eyeballs (see Chapter 18). Medial migration of the eyes from their initial lateral locations results from the enormous growth of the cerebral hemispheres and from the broadening of the head as well as from the real medial movement of the eyes. The greatest migratory movements of the eyes occur from the 5th to 9th weeks post conception; thereafter, they stabilize to the postnatal angulation of the optic axes (at 71° to 68°).

Early in fetal life (8 weeks), folds of surface ectoderm grow over the eyes to form the eyelids (see Fig. 3–10, c and d). These remain fused until the 7th month post conception, when invading muscle allows their opening.

The Ears

The internal ear first manifests as a hindbrain induction of surface ectodermal cells elongating into a thickened otic placode. The placode later invaginates into a pit, which closes off as a vesicle and thus forms the internal ear (see Chapter 18).

The external ear develops in the neck region as six auricular hillocks surrounding the first pharyngeal groove that forms the external acoustic meatus (Fig. 3–12; see also Figs. 3–6 and 3–11). This combination of elevations around a depression forming the auricle appears to rise up the side of the developing face to its ultimate location due to lower facial growth.

The middle ear has a complex origin from the first pharyngeal pouch. Full details of its development are given in Chapter 18.

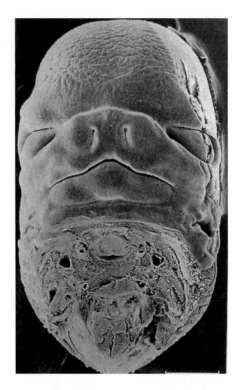

Figure 3–12 Scanning electron micrograph of the face of a 44-day-old human embryo. The merging facial prominences have eliminated the intervening furrows and have diminished the oral opening. The cut surface reveals arteries, veins, the pharynx, and the spinal cord. Auricular hillocks are forming around the external acoustic meatus. (×30 original magnification) (Reproduced with permission from Hinrichson K. The early development of morphology and patterns of the face in the human embryo. In: Advances in anatomy, embryology and cell biology, 98. Springer-Verlag; 1985.)

The Nose

The nose is a complex of contributions from the frontal prominence (the bridge), the merged medial nasal prominences (the median ridge and tip), the lateral nasal prominences (the alae), and the cartilage nasal capsule (the septum and nasal conchae). The internal and external nasal regions develop from two distinct morphogenetic fields: the deep capsular field (giving rise to the cartilaginous nasal capsule and its derivatives) and the superficial alar field (giving rise to the external alar cartilages).

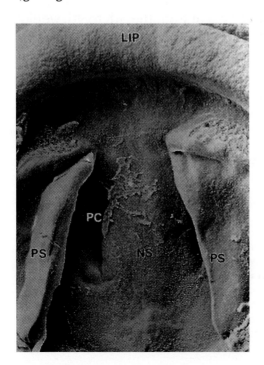

Figure 3–13 Scanning electron micrograph of the stomodeal chamber of a 56-day-old human embryo, revealing the nasal septum (NS) and primary choanae (PC) in the nasal chamber. The palatal shelves (PS) have not yet fused. The upper lip (LIP) is fully fused although the median primary palate has not yet appeared. (×72 original magnification) (Reproduced with permission from Hinrichson K. The early development of morphology and patterns of the face in the human embryo. In: Advances in anatomy, embryology and cell biology, 98. Springer-Verlag; 1985.)

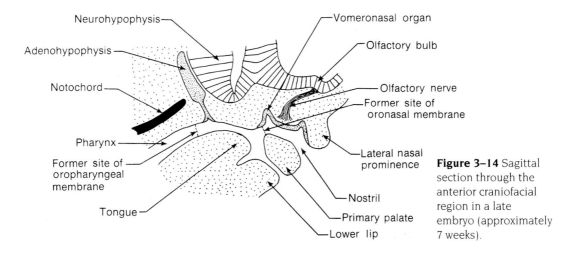

Neurohypophysis

Adenohypophysis

Notochord

Pharynx

Former site of oropharyngeal membrane

Tongue

Vomeronasal organ

Olfactory bulb

Olfactory nerve

Former site of oronasal membrane

Lateral nasal prominence

Nostril

Primary palate

Lower lip

Figure 3–14 Sagittal section through the anterior craniofacial region in a late embryo (approximately 7 weeks).

The nasal pits, previously described, become separated anteriorly from the stomodeum by fusion of the medial nasal, maxillary, and lateral nasal prominences to form the nostrils (anterior nares) (see Fig. 3–12). The blind sacs of the deepening nasal pits are initially separated from the stomodeum by the oronasal membranes that, upon disintegration, establish the primitive posterior nares (primary choanae) (Figs. 3–13 and 3–14). The definitive choanae of the adult are created by fusion of the secondary palatal shelves (described later). While the nostrils become patent early in fetal development, exuberant epithelial growth fills them with plugs until midfetal life.

Within the frontonasal prominence, a mesenchymal condensation forming the precartilaginous nasal capsule develops around the primary nasal cavities as a median mass (the mesethmoid, a prologue to the nasal septum) and paired lateral masses (the ectethmoid) that will form the paired ethmoidal (conchal) and nasal alar cartilages (Fig. 3–15). A cartilaginous nasal floor does not develop in the human. Initially, the primitive nasal septum is a broad area

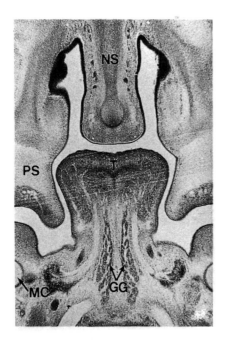

Figure 3–15 Photomicrograph of coronal section of the stomodeum of a 52-day-old human embryo, depicting the vertically oriented palatal shelves (PS) on each side of the tongue (T). Note the nasal septum (NS), genioglossus muscles (GG), and Meckel's cartilage (MC). (Reproduced with permission from O'Rahilly R. A color atlas of human embryology. W. B. Saunders Co.; 1975)

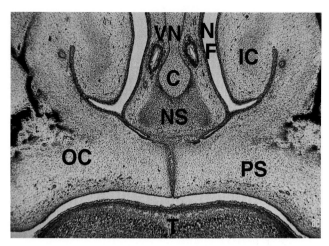

Figure 3–16 Photomicrograph of a coronal section of the palate of a 57-day-old human embryo, depicting fusion of the palatal shelves (PS) with each other and the nasal septum (NS). Epithelial degeneration is seen at the fusion lines. The cartilage (C) of the nasal septum separates the vomeronasal organs (VN). Primary ossification centers (OC) of the maxillae are evident. The inferior conchae (IC) are forming from the ectethmoid. The tongue (T) is separated from the nasal fossae (NF). (Reproduced with permission from O'Rahilly R. A color atlas of human embryology. W. B. Saunders Co.; 1975)

between the primary choanae and never projects as a free process but builds up in a rostrocaudal direction as the later-developing palatal shelves fuse. Within the nasal septum, cartilage forms in continuity with the mesethmoid cartilage, a component of the early basicranium. The nasal septum divides the nasal chamber into left and right fossae; their lateral walls, derived from the ectethmoid, are subdivided into superior, middle, and inferior conchae. The nasal mucosa folds, forming the conchae; these are later invaded by cartilages (Fig. 3–16).

The Vomeronasal Organ

Invasion of ectoderm into the median nasal septum from the nasal fossae between the 6th and 8th weeks forms the bilateral vomeronasal organs (Jacobson's organs), vestigial chemosensory structures (see Fig. 3–16). The

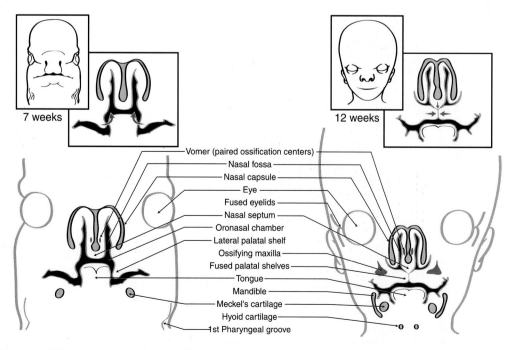

Figure 3–17 Nasal capsule and palate development in coronal section at 7 and 12 weeks post conception.

organs form blind pouches, reaching their fullest development at the 5th month post conception. Thereafter, they diminish and usually disappear but may persist as anomalous cysts and may have a transitory fetal endocrine function. The organ may act as a pheromone receptor in adulthood.

The Nasolacrimal Duct

Within the grooves between the lateral nasal and maxillary prominences, solid rods of epithelial cells sink into the subjacent mesenchyme. The rods, which extend from the developing conjunctival sacs at the medial corners of the forming eyelids to the external nares, later canalize to form the nasolacrimal sacs and ducts. The ducts become completely patent only after birth.

The Early Palate

The primitive stomodeum that forms a wide central shallow depression in the face is limited in its depth by the oropharyngeal membrane. The characteristically deep oral cavity is formed by ventral growth of the prominences surrounding the stomodeum. The stomodeum establishes as an oronasopharyngeal chamber and entrance to the gut on the 28th day, when the dividing oropharyngeal membrane disintegrates, providing continuity of passage between the mouth and pharynx. (The oropharyngeal membrane demarcates the junction of ectoderm and endoderm in the embryo. It is very difficult to trace this line of division subsequently, due to the extensive changes occurring in oropharyngeal development. As the hypophysis originates from Rathke's pouch anterior to the oropharyngeal membrane, a measure of the depth of oral growth is provided by its adult location. The presumed site of the original oropharyngeal membrane in the adult is an imaginary oblique plane from the posterior border of the body of the sphenoid bone through the tonsillar region of the fauces to the sulcus terminalis of the tongue.)

The stomodeal chamber divides into separate oral and nasal cavities when the frontonasal and maxillary prominences develop horizontal extensions into the chamber. These extensions form the central part of the upper lip (the tuberculum), the single median primary palate from the frontonasal prominence, and the two lateral palatal shelves from the maxillary prominences (Fig. 3–17; see also Fig. 3–13). The coincidental development of the tongue from the floor of the mouth fills the oronasal chamber, intervening between the lateral palatal shelves. These shelves are vertically orientated initially but become horizontal when the stomodeum expands and the intervening tongue descends (see Fig. 3–15). The shelves elevate unevenly, with the anterior third "flipping up," followed by an oozing "flow" of the posterior two-thirds.

The elevation of the shelves enables their mutual contact in the midline and their contact with the primary palate anteriorly and the nasal septum superiorly (see Fig. 3–16). Fusion of the shelves, which starts a third of the way from the front, proceeds both anteriorly and posteriorly. The shelves also fuse with the nasal septum, except posteriorly, where the soft palate and uvula remain unattached.

Ossification provides the basis for the anterior bony hard palate. The posterior third of the palate remains unossified; mesenchyme migrates into this

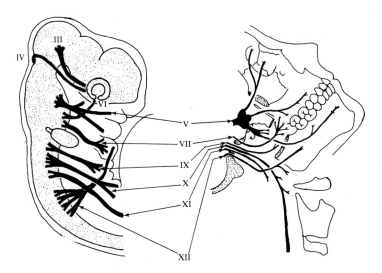

Figure 3–18 Distribution of branches of the cranial nerves in the fetus and adult. III, Oculomotor nerve; IV, trochlear nerve; V, trigeminal nerve; VI abducens nerve; VII, facial nerve; IX, glossopharyngeal nerve; X, vagus nerve; XI, spinal accessory nerve; XII, hypoglossal nerve.

region from the first and fourth pharyngeal arches to provide the soft palate muscles, which retain their initial innervation. (This process is detailed in Chapter 10.)

The Adenohypophysial Pouch

Ectodermal epithelium invaginates upwards in the roof of the primitive stomodeum, immediately ventral to the oropharyngeal membrane, to form the adenohypophysial (Rathke's) pouch and duct (see Fig. 3–7). The location of this diverticulum coincides with the cranial termination of the underlying notochord, and the prechordal mesenchyme is responsible for inducing the diverticulum. This pouch gives rise to the anterior lobe of the pituitary gland (adenohypophysis) by differentiation of the stomodeal ectoderm into endocrine cells; a downward diverticulum of the diencephalon of the forebrain gives rise to the pituitary's posterior lobe (neurohypophysis). Invading neural crest tissue forms the connective-tissue stroma and endocrine cells that produce adrenocorticotropic and melanocyte-stimulating hormones.

The adenohypophysial pouch normally loses contact with the oral ectoderm by atrophy of the hypophysial duct, but remnants may persist within the sphenoid bone as the craniopharyngeal canal. These remnants may become cysts or tumors within the body of the sphenoid bone. Persistent adenohypophysial tissue at the site of origin of the hypophysial duct forms the rare pharyngeal hypophysis.

Seessel's Pouch

A small endodermal diverticulum known as Seessel's pouch develops from the cranial end of the foregut (see Fig. 2–19 in Chapter 2). It arises close to the prechordal plate and projects towards the brain. Seessel's pouch may be represented in the adult by the pharyngeal bursa, a depression in the nasopharyngeal tonsil.

The Oral Cavity

The oral cavity and the entire intestinal tract are sterile at birth. As soon as feeding by mouth commences, an oral bacterial flora that will form part of the oral environment throughout life is established. The oral soft tissues develop a local resistance to infection by this flora, which becomes characteristic of the individual mouth.

The facial contours are expanded in the later stages of fetal development by the formation of a subcutaneous panniculus adiposus, minimal in the scalp and thickest in the cheek. This buccal fat pad minimizes the collapse of the cheeks during suckling. The pale skin of the neonate darkens with melanocyte activity after birth.

DEVELOPMENT OF THE CRANIAL NERVES

Initially, the twelve cranial nerves are organized segmentally and numbered sequentially. This serial pattern is not evident in adulthood, due to the migrations of the nerves' target organs. The tortuous adult nerve pathways trace the embryonic routes of travel of the innervated organs (Fig. 3–18).

The trigeminal (V), facial (VII), and glossopharyngeal (IX) ganglia and parts of the vestibulocochlear (VII) and vagal (X) nerve ganglia derive from the neural crest. Neuroblasts derived from superficial ectodermal placodes in the maxillomandibular region contribute to the ganglia of the trigeminal, facial, vagus, and glossopharyngeal nerves. The surface placodal contributions to these latter nerves may account for the gustatory components. The vestibulo-cochlear ganglion arises from the otic vesicle, neural crest cells, and an ectodermal placode. Caudal to the vagal ganglion, neural crest tissue of the occipital region contributes to ganglia of the accessory (XI) and hypoglossal (XII) nerves.

The central processes of the neurons of these ganglia form the sensory roots of the cranial nerves. Their peripheral processes form the efferent motor components of the nerves.

Sensory innervation of the face by the trigeminal nerve is based upon its embryologic origins. The frontonasal prominence is innervated by the ophthalmic division, the maxillary prominence by the maxillary division, and the mandibular prominence by the mandibular division of the trigeminal nerve. This accounts for the adult pattern of facial sensory innervation, the densest of

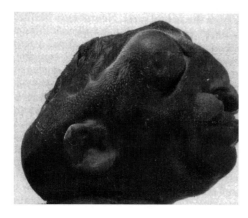

Figure 3–19 Anencephaly, low-set ears, and right cleft lip and palate in an aborted fetus. Note the absence of the calvaria.

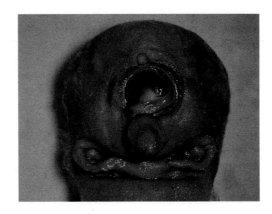

Figure 3–20 An example of combined holoprosencephaly and otocephaly syndromes. Defects include synophthalmia (cyclopia), a median proboscis, synotia, and agnathia.

any cutaneous field. The motor nerve supply is primarily by the facial nerve. (For details, see Chapter 17.)

ANOMALIES OF DEVELOPMENT

Defects of facial development are the result of a multiplicity of etiologic factors, some genetic, most unknown. The study of these anomalies constitutes teratology.

Defective development is categorized into malformations that are generally genetically determined, deformations that are environmentally influenced, and disruptions that are of metabolic, vascular, and/or teratogenic origin. Malformations develop predominantly in the embryonic period and are not self-correcting whereas deformations and disruptions occur in the fetal period and may correct themselves (see Fig. 2–1 in Chapter 2).

The range of facial anomalies is enormous, but all produce some degree of disfigurement and result in the impairment of function to some degree, sometimes even to the point of incompatibility with life. The mechanisms of facial maldevelopment are not well understood, but inductive phenomena arising from the cerebral prosencephalic and rhombencephalic organizing centers are essential to normal facial development. Defective brain development almost inevitably causes cranial or facial dysmorphism.

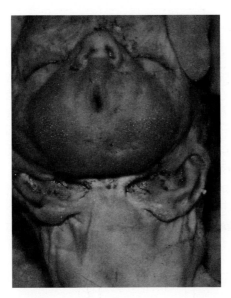

Figure 3–21 A stillborn female 33-week-old fetus with microstomia, aglossia, agnathia, and synotia (otocephalic monster), resulting from aplasia of the first and second pharyngeal arches. (Courtesy of Dr. G. G. Leckie)

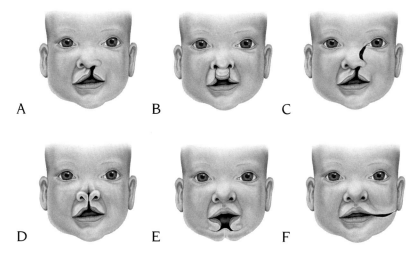

A   B   C

D   E   F

Figure 3–22 Defects of orofacial development: (a) unilateral cleft lip; (b) bilateral cleft lip; (c) oblique facial cleft and cleft lip; (d) median cleft lip and nasal defect; (e) median mandibular cleft; (f) unilateral macrostomia.

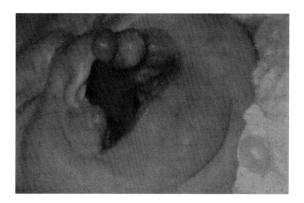

Figure 3–23 Bilateral cleft lip and palate, with consequent projection of the median globular process, in a newborn infant.

Absence of the head (acephaly) is the most extreme defect. Postcranial structures can continue developing in utero; however, the condition is lethal upon birth.

Absence of the brain (anencephaly) results in acrania (absence of the skull), acalvaria (roofless skull), or cranioschisis (fissured cranium), with variable effects upon the face (Fig. 3–19). These fetuses have minimal survival.

Failure of normal telencephalic cleavage of the forebrain into bilateral cerebral hemispheres results in holoprosencephaly, reflecting a disturbed prosencephalic organizing center. This gives rise to a spectrum of upper facial, eye, nose, and ear anomalies, the most severe being cyclopia (synophthalmia) (Fig. 3–20), ranging through ethmocephaly, cebocephaly, premaxillary agenesis (median cleft lip/palate), and premaxillary dysgenesis (bilateral cleft lip/palate) to the mildest dysmorphic manifestation of a single maxillary central incisor tooth. The locations of the eyes, nose, and midmaxilla are variably disturbed, producing a wide assortment of dysmorphic syndromes.

Defects of the rhombencephalic organizing center, which is responsible for induction of the viscerofacial skeleton, account for dysmorphology of the middle and lower thirds of the face (otomandibular syndromes). Defective mandibular development may range from agnathia (absent mandible) associated with ventrally placed cervically located ears (synotia) (Fig. 3–21) to varying degrees of micrognathia and mandibulofacial dysostosis. The rare failure of the mandibular prominences to merge results in mandibular midline cleft.

Mild developmental defects of the face are comparatively common. Failure of the facial prominences to merge or fuse results in abnormal developmental clefts. These clefts are due to the disruption of the many integrated processes of induction, cell migration, local growth, and mesenchymal merging (Fig. 3–22). Bilateral clefting of the upper lip (cheiloschisis) is the result of the medial nasal prominences' failure to merge with the maxillary prominences on either side of the midline (Fig. 3–23). Unilateral cleft lip, more common on the left side, is a relatively common congenital defect (1 in 800 births) that has a strong familial tendency, suggesting a genetic background. The rare bilateral cleft lip results in a wide midline defect of the upper lip and may produce a protuberant mass (Fig. 3–23). The exceedingly rare median cleft lip (the true "hare lip") is due to the incomplete merging of the two medial nasal prominences, therefore leading in most cases (with deep midline grooving of the nose) to various forms of bifid nose.

Merging of the maxillary and mandibular prominences beyond or short of the site for normal mouth size results in a mouth that is too small (microstomia) or too wide (macrostomia) (see Fig. 3–22, f). Microstomial defects are a common feature of syndromes of congenital anomalies of development: trisomy 17 and 18, craniocarpotarsal syndrome (whistling face), otopalatodigital syndrome, and (occasionally) Turner syndrome. Macrostomia occurs in idiopathic hypercalcemia, mandibulofacial dysostosis (Treacher Collins syndrome), and occasionally in Klinefelter's XXY syndrome. Rarely, the maxillary and mandibular prominences fuse, producing a closed mouth (astomia).

An oblique facial cleft results from persistence of the groove between the maxillary prominence and the lateral nasal prominence running from the medial canthus of the eye to the ala of the nose. Persistence of the furrow between the two mandibular prominences produces the rare midline mandibular cleft (see Fig. 3–22, e).

Retardation of mandibular development gives rise to micrognathia of varying degrees, with accompanying dental malocclusion. Total failure of development of the mandible (agnathia) is associated with abnormal ventral placement of the external ears (synotia) (see Fig. 3–21).

Craniofacial developmental cysts, although (strictly speaking) not a defect of orofacial development, originate in the complicated embryonic processes of the craniofacial complex. Developmental cysts arise along the lines of facial and palatal clefts, and their lining epithelia appear to be derived from residues or "rests" of the covering epithelia of the embryonic prominences that merge to form the face. Where such epithelial residues become trapped in the subjacent mesenchyme during merging or where ectopic sequestration of skin or mucosa occurs beneath the surface, there is a potential for cyst formation. In most instances, the subsurface epithelium degenerates, probably by programmed cell death. Persisting epithelial rests may be stimulated to proliferate; after their necrosis, followed by a period of dormancy, they can produce fluid-filled cysts in postnatal life. The nature and cause of stimuli that give rise to these developmental cysts are unknown. These cysts tend to be named according to the site in which they develop; hence, nasolabial cysts develop where the lateral nasal and maxillary prominences meet, globulomaxillary cysts develop more deeply along the line of merging of the median nasal and maxillary prominences, and median mandibular cysts develop in the midline site of the merging of the two mandibular prominences. (Cysts of the pharyngeal arches and palate are dealt with respectively in Chapters 5 and 10.)

Selected Bibliography

Apesos J, Anigian GM. Median cleft of the lip: its significance and surgical repair. Cleft Palate Craniofac J 1993;30:94–6.

Barni T, Fantoni G, Gloria L, et al. Role of endothelin in the human craniofacial morphogenesis. J Craniofac Genet Dev Biol 1998;18:183–94.

Ben Ami M, Weiner E, Perlitz Y, Shalev E. Ultrasound evaluation of the width of the fetal nose. Prenat Diagn 1998;18:1010–13.

Boehm N, Gasser B. Sensory receptor-like cells in the human foetal vomeronasal organ. Neuroreport 1993;4:867–70.

Dattani MT, Robinson IC. The molecular basis for developmental disorders of the pituitary gland in man. Clin Genet 2000;57:337–46.

Diewert VM, Lozanoff S. Growth and morphogenesis of the human embryonic midface during primary palate formation analyzed in frontal sections. J Craniofac Genet Dev Biol 1993;13:162–83.

Diewert VM, Lozanoff S, Choy V. Computer reconstructions of human embryonic craniofacial morphology showing changes in relations between the face and brain during primary palate formation. J Craniofac Genet Dev Biol 1993;13:193–201.

Diewert VM, Shiota K. Morphological observations in normal primary palate and cleft lip embryos in the Kyoto collection. Teratology 1990;41:663–77.

Diewert VM, Wang KY. Recent advances in primary palate and midface morphogenesis research. Crit Rev Oral Biol Med 1992;4:111–30.

Garrosa M, Gayoso MJ, Esteban FJ. Prenatal development of the mammalian vomeronasal organ. Microsc Res Tech 1998;41:456–70.

Hu D, Helms JA. The role of sonic hedgehog in normal and abnormal craniofacial morphogenesis. Development 1999;126:4873–84.

Johnson MC, Bronsky PT. Prenatal craniofacial development: new insights on normal and abnormal mechanisms. Crit Rev Oral Biol Med 1995;6:368–422.

Kehrli P, Maillot C, Wolff MJ. Anatomy and embryology of the trigeminal nerve and its branches in the parasellar area. Neurol Res 1997;19:57–65.

Kjaer I, Fischer-Hansen B. Human fetal pituitary gland in holoprosencephaly and anencephaly. J Craniofac Genet Dev Biol 1995;15:222–9.

Kjaer I, Fischer-Hansen B. The human vomeronasal organ: prenatal developmental stages and distribution of luteinizing hormone-releasing hormone. Eur J Oral Sci 1996;104:34–40.

Kosaka K, Hama K, Eto K. Light and electron microscopy study of fusion of facial prominences. A distinctive type of superficial cells at the contact sites. Anat Embryol 1985;173:187–201.

Lekkas C, Latief BS, Corputty JE. Median cleft of the lower lip associated with lip pits and cleft of the lip and palate. Cleft Palate Craniofac J 1998;35:269–71.

Martin RA, Jones KL, Benirschke K. Extension of the cleft lip phenotype: the subepithelial cleft. Am J Med Genet 1993;47:744–7.

Mooney MP, Siegel MI, Kimes KR, Todhunter J. Premaxillary development in normal and cleft lip and palate human fetuses using three-dimensional computer reconstruction. Cleft Palate Craniofac J 1991;28:49–54.

Namnoum JD, Hisley KC, Graepel S, et al. Three-dimensional reconstruction of the human fetal philtrum. Ann Plast Surg 1997;38:202–8.

Oostrom CA, Vermeij-Keers C, Gilbert PM, van der Meulen JC. Median cleft of the lower lip and mandible: case reports, a new embryologic hypothesis, and subdivision. Plast Reconstr Surg 1996;97:313–20.

Pretorius DH, Nelson TR. Fetal face visualization using three-dimensional ultrasonography. J Ultrasound Med 1995;14:349–56.

Richman JM. Head development. Craniofacial genetics makes headway. Curr Biol 1995;5:345–8.

Sataloff RT. Embryology of the facial nerve and its clinical applications. Laryngoscope 1990;100:969–84.

Sherwood RJ, McLachlan JC, Aiton JF, Scarborough J. The vomeronasal organ in the human embryo, studied by means of three-dimensional computer reconstruction. J Anat 1999;195:413–8.

Siegel MI, Mooney MP, Kimes KR, Todhunter J. Developmental correlates of midfacial components in a normal and cleft lip and palate human fetal sample. Cleft Palate Craniofac J 1991;28:408–12.

Smith TD, Siegel MI, Mooney MP, et al. Vomeronasal organ growth and development in normal and cleft lip and palate human fetuses. Cleft Palate Craniofac J 1996;33:385–94.

Smith TD, Siegel MI, Mooney MP, et al. Prenatal growth of the human vomeronasal organ. Anat Rec 1997;248:447–55.

Sulik KK. Dr. Beverly R. Rollnick memorial lecture. Normal and abnormal craniofacial embryogenesis. Birth Defects Orig Artic Ser 1990;26:1–18.

Sulik KK, Schoenwolf GC. Highlights of craniofacial morphogenesis in mammalian embryos, as revealed by scanning electron microscopy. Scan Electron Microsc 1985;(Pt 4):1735–52.

Thorogood P, Ferretti P. Heads and tales: recent advances in craniofacial development. Br Dent J 1992;173:301–6.

Varga ZM, Wegner J, Westerfield M. Anterior movement of ventral diencephalic precursors separates the primordial eye field in the neural plate and requires cyclops. Development 1999;126:5533–46.

Williams A, Pizzuto M, Brodsky L, Perry R. Supernumerary nostril: a rare congenital deformity. Int J Pediatr Otorhinolaryngal 1998;44:161–7.

Wyszynski DF, editor. Cleft lip and palate: from origin to treatment. New York: Oxford University Press; 2001. [In press].

Zbar RIS, Zbar LIS, Dudley C, et al. A classification scheme for the vomeronasal organ in humans. Plast Reconstr Surg 2000;105:1284–8.

4 PHARYNGEAL ARCHES

Starting from a single cell, I passed one period of my life with gill slits inherited from my fishy ancestry, then for a few weeks sported a tail and was hard to distinguish from an unborn tree shrew....Why think of viruses or pre-Cambrian organisms, when inside this delicate membrane of my skin, this outline of an individual, I carry the whole history of life.

Jaquetta Hawkes, 1953

NORMAL DEVELOPMENT

During the late somite period (4th week post conception), the mesoderm lateral plate of the ventral foregut region becomes segmented to form a series of five distinct bilateral mesenchyme swellings called the pharyngeal (branchial) arches. Ventrally migrating neural crest cells interact with lateral extensions of the pharyngeal endoderm, surround the six aortic arch arteries, and initiate pharyngeal arch development. The initial mesodermal core of each arch is augmented by neural crest tissue that surrounds the mesodermal core.

Figure 4–1 Schematic diagram of embryo, with sectioned pharyngeal arches.

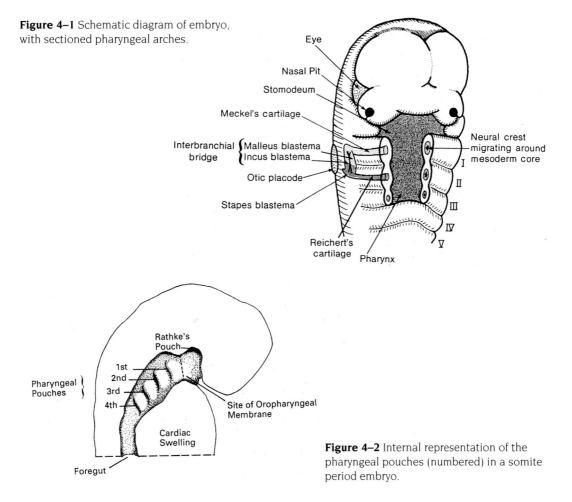

Figure 4–2 Internal representation of the pharyngeal pouches (numbered) in a somite period embryo.

The mesoderm will give rise to muscle myoblasts while the neural crest cells give rise to skeletal and connective tissues.

The pharyngeal arches are separated by pharyngeal grooves on the external aspect of the embryo, which correspond internally with five outpouchings of the elongated pharynx of the foregut, known as the five pharyngeal pouches (Figs. 4–1 and 4–2). Although derivatives of five or even six arches are described, only three (and exceptionally, four) arches appear externally. Caudal to the third arch, there is a depression, the cervical sinus.

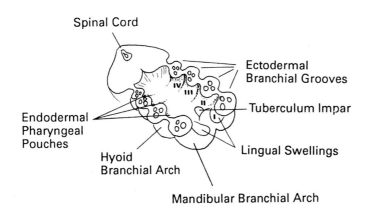

Figure 4–3 Schema of early pharyngeal arch development. Pharyngeal arches are numbered in Roman numerals. (After Waterman and Meller) (Reproduced with permission from Shaw JH, Sweeney EA, Cappuccino CC, Meller SM. Textbook of oral biology. Philadelphia: W.B. Saunders; 1978.)

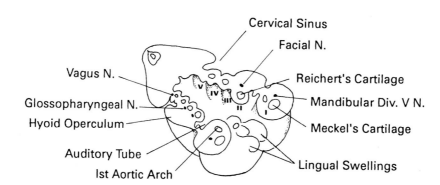

Figure 4–4 Schema of lateral pharyngeal arch development. Pharyngeal arches are numbered in Roman numerals. V, fifth cranial nerve; N, nerve. (After Waterman and Meller) (Reproduced with permission from Shaw JH, Sweeney EA, Cappuccino CC, Meller SM. Textbook of oral biology. Philadelphia: W.B. Saunders; 1978.)

The pharyngeal arches decrease in size from cranial to caudal, each pair merging midventrally to form "collars" in the cervical region. Each of the five pairs of arches contains the following basic set of structures (Figs. 4–3 to 4–6; Table 4–1):

1. A central cartilage rod that forms the skeleton of the arch
2. A muscular component
3. A vascular component (an aortic arch artery) that runs around the pharynx from the ventrally located heart to the dorsal aorta
4. A nervous element consisting of sensory and special visceral motor fibers of one or more cranial nerves supplying the mucosa and muscle arising from that arch

TABLE 4–1 Derivatives of the Pharyngeal System

Pharyngeal Arch	Ectodermal Groove	Endodermal Pouch	Skeleton	Viscera	Artery	Muscles	Motor Nerve	Sensory Nerve
1st (mandibular)	Ext acoustic meatus: ear hillocks; pinna	Auditory tube; middle-ear tympanum	Meckel's cartilage: malleus; incus (mandible template)	Body of tongue	Ext carotid artery Maxillary artery	Masticatory, tensor tympani, mylohyoid, ant digastric	Mandibular division of V: trigeminal	V: lingual nerve
2nd (hyoid)	Disappears	Tonsillar fossa	Reichert's cartilage Stapes, styloid process; sup hyoid body	Midtongue: thyroid gland anlage; tonsil	Stapedial artery (disappears)	Facial, stapedius, stylohyoid postdigastric	VII: facial	VII: chorda tympani
3rd	Disappears	Inf parathyroid 3; thymus	Inf hyoid body, greater cornu hyoid	Root of tongue: fauces; epiglottis; thymus Inf parathyroid 3 Carotid body	Int carotid artery	Stylopharyngeus	IX: glossopharyngeal	IX: glossopharyngeal
4th	Disappears	Sup parathyroid 4	Thyroid and laryngeal cartilages	Pharynx: epiglottis Sup parathyroid 4 Para-aortic bodies	Aorta (L) Subclavian (R)	Pharyngeal constrictors Levator palatini Palatoglossus Palatopharyngeus Cricothyroid	X: superior laryngeal nerve (vagus)	X: auricular nerve to ext acoustic meatus
6th	Disappears	Telopharyngeal (ultimopharyngeal) body (cyst) Calcitonin "C" cells	Cricoid, arytenoid, corniculate cartilages	Larynx	Pulmonary arteries Ductus arteriosus	Laryngeal, pharyngeal constrictors	X: inferior laryngeal nerve (vagus)	X: vagus
Postpharyngeal region somites 4 occipital somites			Tracheal cartilages SCLEROTOMES Basioccipital bone			Trapezius: sternomastoid MYOTOMIC MUSCLE Intrinsic tongue muscles Styloglossus Hyoglossus Genioglossus } Exterior tongue muscles	XI: spinal accessory XII: hypoglossal	
Prechordal somites			Nasal capsule Nasal septum		Extrinsic ocular		III: oculomotor IV: trochlear VI: abducens	
Upper cervical somites			Cervical vertebrae		Geniohyoid; infrahyoid		Spinal nerves C1, somites C2	

ant = anterior; ext = exterior; inf = inferior; int = interior; L = left; post = posterior; R = right; sup = superior.

The cartilage rods, which are differentiated from neural crest tissue that has been organized by pharyngeal endoderm, are variously adapted to bony, cartilaginous, or ligamentous structures. In some cases, the rods disappear in later development. The muscle components are of somitomeric and somitic origin and give rise to special visceral muscles composed of striated muscle fibers. Nerve fibers of specific cranial nerves enter the mesoderm of the pharyngeal arches, initiating muscle development in the mesoderm. The muscles arising from the mesodermal cores migrate from their sites of origin and adapt to the pharyngeal arch derivatives. The original nerve supply to these muscles is maintained during migration, accounting for the devious routes of many cranial nerves in adults. The vascular system originates from lateral plate mesoderm and neural crest tissue angioblasts. The arteries are modified from their symmetric primitive embryonic pattern to the asymmetric form of the adult derivatives of the fourth and sixth arch arteries (see Table 4–1).

First Pharyngeal Arch

The first (or mandibular) pharyngeal arch is the precursor of both the maxillary and mandibular jaws and appropriately bounds the lateral aspects of the stomodeum, which is merely a depression in the early facial region at this stage. The maxilla is derived from a small maxillary prominence extending cranioventrally from the much larger mandibular prominence derived from the first arch. The cartilage skeleton of the first arch, known as Meckel's cartilage (see Fig. 4–1), arises at the 41st to 45th days post conception and provides a template for subsequent development of the mandible; however, most of its cartilage substance disappears in the formed mandible. The mental ossicle is the only portion of the mandible derived from Meckel's cartilage by endochondral ossification.

Persisting portions of Meckel's cartilage form the basis of major portions of two ear ossicles: (1) the head and neck of the malleus (the anterior process of the malleus forms independently in membrane bone [os goniale]); (2) the body and short crus of the incus (the incus arises from the separated dorsal end of Meckel's cartilage that corresponds to the pterygoquadrate cartilage of inframammalian vertebrates); and (3) two ligaments—the anterior ligament of the malleus and the sphenomandibular ligament. The musculature of the mandibular arch, originating from cranial somitomere 4, subdivides and migrates to form the muscles of mastication, the mylohyoid muscle, the anterior belly of the digastric, the tensor tympani (the evolutionary remnant of a reptilian jaw muscle attached to the remnant of the reptilian jaw [ie, Meckel's cartilage]), and the tensor veli palatini muscles, all of which are innervated by the nerve of the first arch (the mandibular division of the fifth cranial, or trigeminal, nerve) (see Fig. 4–4). The sensory component of this nerve innervates the mandible and its covering mucosa and gingiva, the mandibular teeth, the mucosa of the anterior two-thirds of the tongue, the floor of the mouth, and the skin of the lower third of the face. The first-arch artery contributes in part to the maxillary artery and part of the external carotid artery.

Second Pharyngeal Arch

The cartilage of the second (or hyoid) arch (Reichert's cartilage) appears on the 45th to 48th days post conception. It is the basis of the greater part (head, neck, and crura) of the third ear ossicle (the stapes*) and contributes to the malleus and incus,† the styloid process of the temporal bone, the stylohyoid ligament, and the lesser horn and cranial part of the body of the hyoid bone (Fig. 4–7). Reichert's cartilage attaches to the basicranial otic capsule, where it is grooved by the facial nerve; it provides the remaining cartilaginous circumference to the labyrinthine and tympanic segments of the facial canal.

The muscles of the hyoid arch originating from cranial somitomere 6 subdivide and migrate extensively to form the stapedius, the stylohyoid, the posterior belly of the digastric, and the mimetic muscles of the face, all of which are innervated by the seventh cranial (or *facial*) nerve, serving the second arch. The paths of migration of these muscles are traced out in the adult by the distribution of branches of the facial nerve. This nerve's special sensory component for taste, known as the chorda tympani, invades the first arch as a pretrematic nerve and thus comes to supply the mucosa of the anterior two-thirds of the tongue. The artery of this arch forms the stapedial artery, which disappears during the fetal period, leaving the foramen in the stapes. (A branch of

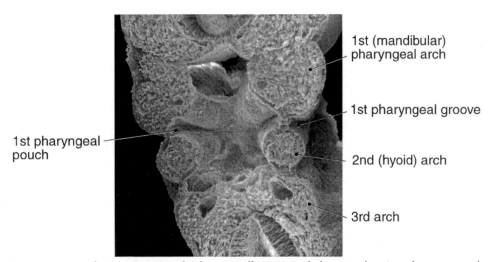

Figure 4–5 Scanning electron micrograph of a coronally sectioned pharyngeal region of a mouse embryo corresponding to an approximately 28-day-old human embryo. (Courtesy of Dr. K. K. Sulik)

the internal carotid artery, the stapedial artery, initially supplies the deep portion of the face, an area that is taken over by branches of the external carotid artery once the stapedial artery disappears.)

The stapedial artery, derived from the second aortic arch, is significant in the development of the stapes ear ossicle. The stapedial blastema grows around the stapedial artery, forming a ring around the centrally placed artery. The midportion of the stapedial artery involutes, leaving the foramen in the stapes. Stapedial arterial branches persist, to become part of the internal carotid artery proximally and the external carotid artery distally.

---

*The first ossicle to appear. The footplate (base) of the stapes is derived in part from the lateral wall of the otic capsule.
†The manubrium of the malleus and the long crus of the incus are derived from the interpharyngeal bridge, which arises from the second arch.

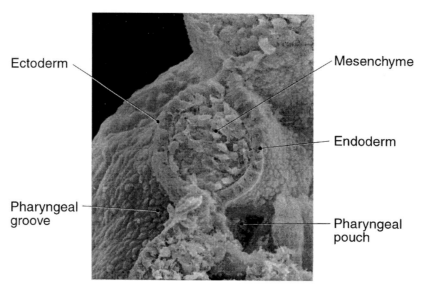

Figure 4–6 Magnified scanning electron micrograph of a coronally sectioned pharyngeal arch of a 9-day-old mouse embryo corresponding to a 28-day-old human embryo. Details of cellular components are shown. (Courtesy of Dr. K. K. Sulik)

Third Pharyngeal Arch

The cartilage of this small arch produces the greater horn (cornu) and the caudal part of the body of the hyoid bone. The remainder of the cartilage disappears. The mesoderm originating from cranial somitomere 7 forms the stylopharyngeus muscle, innervated by the ninth cranial (or *glossopharyngeal*) nerve supplying the arch. The mucosa of the posterior third of the tongue is derived from this arch, accounting for its sensory innervation by the glossopharyngeal nerve.

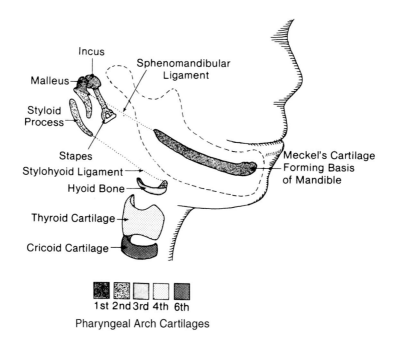

Figure 4–7 Derivatives of the pharyngeal arch cartilages. Note that the malleus, incus, and hyoid bones are each derived from two pharyngeal arches.

The artery of this arch contributes to the common carotid and part of the internal carotid arteries. Neural crest tissue in the third arch forms the carotid body, which first appears as a mesenchymal condensation around the third aortic arch artery. This chemoreceptor body thus derives its nerve supply from the glossopharyngeal nerve.

Fourth Pharyngeal Arch

The cartilage of the fourth pharyngeal arch probably forms the thyroid cartilage. The arch muscles originating from occipital somites 2 and 4 develop into the cricothyroid and constrictors of the pharynx, the palatopharyngeus, levator veli palatini and uvular muscles of the soft palate, and the palatoglossus muscle of the tongue. The nerve of the fourth arch is the superior laryngeal branch of the 10th cranial (or vagus) nerve, which innervates these muscles.

The fourth-arch artery of the left side forms the arch of the aorta; that of the right side contributes to the right subclavian and brachiocephalic arteries. The para-aortic bodies of chromaffin cells that secrete noradrenalin arise from the ectomesenchyme of the fourth and sixth pharyngeal arches.

Fifth Pharyngeal Arch

The fifth arch, a transitory structure, disappears almost as soon as it forms. It bequeaths no permanent structural elements.

Sixth Pharyngeal Arch

The cartilage of the sixth arch probably forms the cricoid and arytenoid cartilages of the larynx. The mesoderm originating from occipital somites 1 and 2 forms the intrinsic muscles of the larynx, which are supplied by the nerve of the arch, the recurrent laryngeal branch of the vagus nerve. Because the nerve of this arch passes caudal to the fourth-arch artery in its recurring path from the brain to the muscles it supplies, the differing fate of the left and right fourth-arch arteries, when they migrate caudally into the thorax, accounts for the different recurrent paths of the left and right laryngeal nerves. The right recurrent laryngeal nerve recurves around the right subclavian artery (derived from the fourth-arch artery); the left laryngeal nerve recurves around the aorta (also derived from the fourth-arch artery), due to the disappearance of the dorsal part of the sixth aortic artery and all of the fifth aortic artery.

Parts of the sixth-arch arteries develop into the pulmonary arteries; the remaining parts on the right side disappear, and those on the left side form the temporary ductus arteriosus of the fetus. This later becomes the ligamentum arteriosum.

Postpharyngeal Region

Controversy surrounds the embryologic origin of the tracheal cartilages and the sternomastoid and trapezius muscles. On the basis of their nerve supply (spinal accessory [11th cranial] nerve), it appears that the latter two muscles are of mixed somitic and pharyngeal-arch origin.

The Hyoid Bone

The hyoid bone, a composite endochondral bone derived from the cartilages of the second (hyoid) and third pharyngeal arches, reflects its double ori-

TABLE 4–2 Possible Anomalies of the Pharyngeal System

Pharyngeal Arch	Ectodermal Groove	Endodermal Pouch	Skeleton	Artery	Muscles	Nerve
1st (mandibular)	Aplasia, atresia, stenosis, duplication of ext acoustic meatus	Diverticulum of auditory tube; aplasia, atresia, stenosis of tube	Aplasia/dysplasia of malleus, incus, mandible	Hypoplastic/absent ext carotid and maxillary arteries	Deficient masticatory/facial muscles	Absent mandibular nerve
2nd (hyoid)	Cervical (pharyngeal) cleft, sinus, cyst, fistula	Tonsillar sinus, pharyngeal fistula	Aplasia/dysplasia of stapes, styloid process	Persistent stapedial artery	Deficient facial, stapedial muscles	Deficient facial, chorda tympani nerve
3rd	Cervical cleft, sinus, cyst, fistula	Cervical thymus: thymic cyst; aplasia parathyroid 3; aplasia thymus (DiGeorge anomaly)	Defective hyoid bone	Hypoplastic/absent int carotid artery		Deficient glossopharyngeal nerve
4th	Cervical cleft, sinus, cyst, fistula	Fistula/sinus from pyriform sinus; aplasia parathyroid 4	Congenital laryngeal stenosis, cleft, atresia (Fraser's syndrome)	Double aortae: aortic interruption; right aorta	Deficient faucial muscles	Deficient vagus nerve
6th		Aplasia of calcitonin parafollicular cells (DiGeorge anomaly)		Aorticopulmonary septation anomalies (DiGeorge anomaly)		

ext = exterior; int = interior.

gin in its six centers of ossification, two for the body and one for each lesser and each greater horn.* Ossification centers for the greater horns appear at the end of fetal life (38 weeks), those for the body appear at about birth, and those for the lesser horns appear about 2 years after birth. The lesser horns may not fuse with the body but attach by fibrous tissue to the greater horns, which in turn articulate with the body through a diarthrodial synovial joint. The double origin of the hyoid body (from the second and third arches) is very occasionally reflected as a split into upper and lower portions. The fusion of all these elements into a single bone occurs in early childhood.

ANOMALIES OF DEVELOPMENT

Deficient development of the pharyngeal arches results in syndromes that are identified according to the arch(es) involved (first-arch syndrome, second-arch syndrome, etc.), becoming rarer as the number of the arch increases, and reflecting deficiencies of all or some of the derivatives of that arch. Examples of severe first-arch anomalies are agnathia, synotia, and microstomia. Less-severe anomalies are mandibulofacial dysostosis (Treacher Collins syndrome) and micrognathia combined with cleft palate (Pierre Robin syndrome). External-ear deficiencies (anotia and microtia), auricular tags, and persistent pharyngeal clefts or cysts (auricular sinuses) are among the more common examples of pharyngeal-arch anomalies.

Anomalies of the second and subsequent arches involve the hyoid (laryngeal) apparatus and are very rare. Mineralization of the stylohyoid ligament elongates the styloid process and may cause craniocervical pain, dysphagia, odynophagia, and foreign-body discomfort of the pharynx (Eagle syndrome). The condition may be inherited by an autosomal dominant gene on chromosome 6p (Table 4–2).

Selected Bibliography

Bamforth JS, Machin GA. Severe hemifacial microsomia and absent right pharyngeal arch artery derivatives in a 19-week-old fetus. Birth Defects Orig Artic Ser 1996;30(1):227–45.

Caton A, Hacker A, Naeem A, et al. The branchial arches and HGF are growth-promoting and chemoattractant for cranial motor axons. Development 2000;127:1751–66.

Clementi M, Mammi I, Tenconi R. Family with branchial arch anomalies, hearing loss, ear and commissural lip pits, and rib anomalies. A new autosomal recessive condition: branchio-oto-costal syndrome? Am J Med Genet 1997;68:91–3.

Ferguson CA, Tucker AS, Sharpe PT. Temporospatial cell interactions regulating mandibular and maxillary arch patterning. Development 2000;127:403–12.

---

*The hyoid bone consists of several independent elements that, although fused together in man, remain separate in many animals as the "hyoid apparatus." Of these separate elements, the tympanohyal and stylohyal form the styloid process in humans. The ceratohyal forms the lesser horn and upper part of the body of the human hyoid. The epihyal does not form a bone in humans but is incorporated into the stylohyoid ligament. The thyrohyal that develops from the third arch forms the greater horn and lower part of the body of the human hyoid bone.

Gavalas A, Studer M, Lumsden A, et al. Hoxa1 and Hoxb1 synergize in patterning the hindbrain, cranial nerves and second pharyngeal arch. Development 1998;125:1123–36.

Hunt P, Whiting J, Muchamore I, et al. Homeobox genes and models for patterning the hindbrain and branchial arches. Development Suppl 1991;1:187–96.

Jacobsson C, Granstrom G. Clinical appearance of spontaneous and induced first and second branchial arch syndromes. Scand J Plast Reconstr Surg Hand Surg 1997;31:125–36.

Kruchinskii GV. Classification of the syndromes of branchial arches 1 and 2. Acta Chir Plast 1990;32:178–90.

Merida-Velasco JA, Sanchez-Montesinos I, Espin-Ferra J, et al. Ectodermal ablation of the third branchial arch in chick embryos and the morphogenesis of the parathyroid III gland. J Craniofac Genet Dev Biol 1999;9:33–40.

Pearl WR. Single arterial trunk arising from the aortic arch. Evidence that the fifth branchial arch can persist as the definitive aortic arch. Pediatr Radiol 1991;21:518–20.

Pretterklieber ML, Krammer EB. Sphenoidal artery, ramus orbitalis persistens and pterygospinosus muscle —a unique cooccurrence of first branchial arch anomalies in man. Acta Anat 1996;155:136–44.

Qiu M, Bulfone A, Ghattas I, et al. Role of the Dlx homeobox genes in proximodistal patterning of the branchial arches: mutations of Dlx-1. Dev Biol 1997;185:164–84.

Stratakis CA, Lin JP, Rennert OM. Description of a large kindred with autosomal dominant inheritance of branchial arch anomalies, hearing loss, and ear pits, and exclusion of the branchio-oto-renal (BOR) syndrome gene locus (chromosome 8q13.3). Am J Med Genet 1998;79:209–14.

Tucker AS, Yamada G, Grigoriou M, et al. Fgf-8 determines rostral-caudal polarity in the first branchial arch. Development 1999;126:51–61.

Veitch E, Begbie J, Schilling F, et al. Pharyngeal arch patterning in the absence of neural crest. Curr Biol 1999;9:1481–4.

Vieille-Grosjean I, Hunt P, Gulisano M, et al. Branchial HOX gene expression and human craniofacial development. Dev Biol 1997;183:49–60.

Whitworth IH, Suvarna SK, Wight RG, Walsh-Waring GP. Fourth branchial arch anomaly: a rare incidental finding in an adult. J Laryngol Otol 1993;107:238–9.

5 PHARYNGEAL POUCHES AND PHARYNGEAL GROOVES

NORMAL DEVELOPMENT

The primitive pharynx forms in the late embryonic period as a dilation of the cranial end of the foregut, lying between the developing heart ventrally and the developing chondrocranium rostrodorsally. The early pharynx is large relative to the rest of the gut, is flattened ventrodorsally, and gives rise to diverse structures from its floor and side walls. The lateral aspects of the comparatively elongated primitive pharynx project a series of pouches between the pharyngeal arches. These pharyngeal pouches sequentially decrease in size craniocaudally (Fig. 5–1). Intervening between the pharyngeal arches

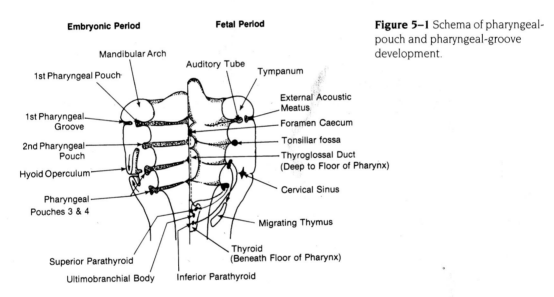

Figure 5–1 Schema of pharyngeal-pouch and pharyngeal-groove development.

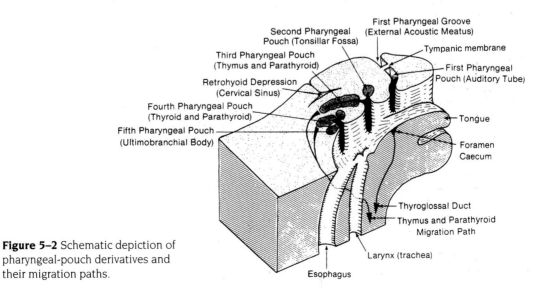

Figure 5–2 Schematic depiction of pharyngeal-pouch derivatives and their migration paths.

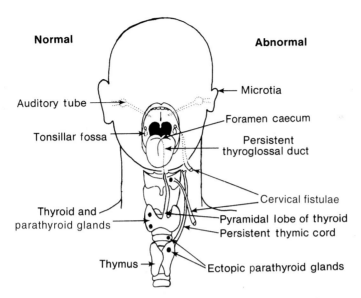

Normal   **Abnormal**

Auditory tube

Tonsillar fossa

Thyroid and
parathyroid glands

Thymus →

Microtia

Foramen caecum

Persistent
thyroglossal duct

Cervical fistulae

Pyramidal lobe of thyroid

Persistent thymic cord

Ectopic parathyroid glands

Figure 5–3 Adult normal
and anomalous derivatives
of pharyngeal pouches.

externally are the pharyngeal grooves (ectodermal clefts) (see Figs. 4–1, 4–3, and 4–4 in Chapter 4). The lining of the pharyngeal grooves is the surface ectoderm; that of the internal pharyngeal pouches is foregut endoderm. Each ectodermal pharyngeal groove corresponds with each endodermal pharyngeal pouch, with a layer of mesodermal mesenchyme intervening between the outer and inner primary germ layers.

The endodermal lining of the primitive pharynx develops gradually from a polyhedral cuboidal embryonic epithelium into a respiratory mucous membrane characterized by goblet cells and a ciliated columnar epithelium.

The first pharyngeal groove persists, and while its ventral end is obliterated, its dorsal end deepens to form the external acoustic meatus. The ectomesoendodermal membrane in the depth of the groove, separating it from the first pharyngeal pouch, persists as the tympanic membrane (Fig. 5–2). (Subsequent external- and middle-ear development is described in Chapter 18.)

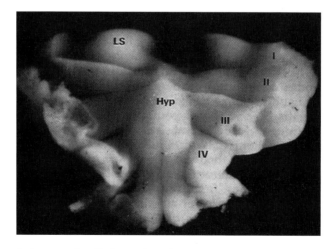

Figure 5–4 The ventral pharyngeal wall of a 32-day-old embryo. The pharyngeal arches are marked I to IV. The lingual swellings (LS) are rising from the first pharyngeal arches. The hypopharyngeal eminence (Hyp) forms a prominent central elevation from which the epiglottis will arise. (×41 original magnification) (Courtesy of Professor H. Nishimura)

The second, third, and fourth pharyngeal grooves become obliterated by the caudal overgrowth of the second pharyngeal arch (hyoid operculum), which provides a smooth contour to the neck. At the end of the 5th week post conception, the third and fourth pharyngeal arches are collectively sunk into a retrohyoid depression, the cervical sinus. The failure of these pharyngeal grooves to be obliterated completely results in a pharyngeal fistula leading from the pharynx to the outside or in a pharyngeal (cervical) sinus or cyst, forming a closed sac (Fig 5–3). Most pharyngeal cysts and fistulae originate from the second groove. If derived from the pharyngeal pouch, they are lined by columnar or ciliated epithelium; if from the pharyngeal groove, they are lined by squamous epithelium.

Thickened ectodermal epibranchial placodes develop at the dorsal ends of the first, second, and fourth pharyngeal grooves. These placodes contribute to the ganglia of the facial, glossopharyngeal, and vagus nerves (see p. 44).

The five pairs of pharyngeal pouches on the sides of the pharyngeal foregut form dorsal and ventral pockets, the endodermal epithelium of which differentiates into various structures. Elongation of the third, fourth, and fifth pharyngeal pouches during the 6th and 7th weeks post conception increasingly dissociates the pouches from the pharynx, allowing their derivatives to form in the lower anterior neck region (Fig. 5–4 and Table 4–1 in Chapter 4; see also Figs. 5–1 and 5–2).

First Pharyngeal Pouch

The ventral portion of the first pouch is obliterated by the developing tongue. The dorsal diverticulum deepens laterally as the tubotympanic recess to form the auditory tube, widening at its end into the tympanum, or middle-ear cavity, and separated from the first pharyngeal groove by the tympanic membrane (see Figs. 5–1 and 5–2). The tympanum becomes occupied by the dorsal ends of the cartilages of the first and second pharyngeal arches that develop into the ear ossicles. The tympanum maintains contact with the pharynx via the auditory tube throughout life.

The proximal portion of the expanding and elongating auditory tube becomes lined with respiratory mucous membrane, and fibrous tissue and cartilage form in its walls. In the 4th month post conception, chondrification occurs from four centers in the adjacent mesoderm. Growth of the cartilaginous portion of the tube is greatest between 16 and 28 weeks post conception. Thereafter, the increase in tubal length is primarily in the osseous portion of the tube. The changing location of the opening of the auditory tube reflects the growth of the nasopharynx. The tubal orifice is inferior to the hard palate in the fetus, is level with it at birth, and is well above the hard palate in the adult.

Second Pharyngeal Pouch

The ventral portion of the second pouch is also obliterated by the developing tongue. The dorsal portion of this pouch persists in an attenuated form as the tonsillar fossa, the endodermal lining of which covers the underlying mesodermal lymphatic tissue to form the palatine tonsil. (Note that neither the pharyngeal nor the lingual tonsils originate from the pharyngeal pouch.)

Third Pharyngeal Pouch

The ventral diverticulum endoderm proliferates and migrates from each side to form two elongated diverticula that grow caudally into the surrounding mesenchyme to form the elements of the thymus gland. The two thymic rudiments meet in the midline but do not fuse, being united by connective tissue. Lymphoid cells invade the thymus from hemopoietic tissue during the 3rd month post conception.

The dorsal diverticulum endoderm differentiates and then migrates caudally to form the inferior parathyroid gland (parathyroid 3). The glands derived from the endodermal lining of the pouch lose their connection with the pharyngeal wall when the pouches become obliterated during later development. The lateral glossoepiglottic fold represents the third pharyngeal pouch.

Fourth Pharyngeal Pouch

The fate of the endoderm of the ventral diverticulum is uncertain; the lining membrane may contribute to thymus or thyroid tissue.

The dorsal diverticulum endoderm differentiates into the superior parathyroid gland (parathyroid 4), which after losing contact with the pharynx, migrates caudally with the thyroid gland. The aryepiglottic fold represents the fourth pharyngeal pouch.

Fifth Pharyngeal Pouch

The attenuated fifth pharyngeal pouch appears as a diverticulum of the fourth pouch. The endoderm of the fifth pouch forms the ultimopharyngeal body. The calcitonin-secreting cells of this structure, however, are derived from neural crest tissue and are eventually incorporated into the thyroid gland as parafollicular cells. The laryngeal ventricles could represent the remnants of the fifth pharyngeal pouch.

ANOMALIES OF DEVELOPMENT

Defective development of the pharyngeal pouches results in defects of their derivatives (see Fig 5–3). The most common anomalies are pharyngeal fistulae and cysts and persistent tracks of migrated glands derived from the pouches. Atresia of the auditory tube is rare. Congenital absence of the thymus and parathyroid glands (and thus, of their products) results in metabolic defects and increased susceptibility to infection (DiGeorge syndrome). Other possible anomalies are listed in Table 4–1 in Chapter 4.

Selected Bibliography

Atlan G, Egerszegi EP, Brochu P, et al. Cervical chondrocutaneous branchial remnants. Plast Reconstr Surg 1997;100:32–9.

Begbie J, Brunet JF, Rubenstein JL, Graham A. Induction of the epibranchial placodes. Development 1999;126:895–902.

Bluestone CD. The eustachian tube. Toronto: B.C. Decker Inc.; 2000.

Fraser BA, Duckworth JWA. Ultimobranchial body cysts in the human foetal thyroid: pathological implications. J Pathol 1979;127:89–92.

Hickey SA, Scott GA, Traub P. Defects of the first branchial cleft. J Laryngol Otol 1994;108:240–3.

Johnson IJ, Soames JV, Birchall JP. Fourth branchial arch fistula. J Laryngol Otol 1996;110:391–3.

Nofsinger YC, Tom LW, LaRossa D, et al. Periauricular cysts and sinuses. Laryngoscope 1997;107:883–7.

Scheuerle AE, Good RA, Habal MB. Involvement of the thymus and cellular immune system in craniofacial malformation syndromes. J Craniofac Surg 1990; 1:88–90.

Sperber GH, Sperber SM. Pharyngogenesis. J Dent Assoc South Africa 1996; 51:777–82.

Vade A, Griffiths A, Hotaling A, et al. Thymopharyngeal duct cyst: MR imaging of a third branchial arch anomaly in a neonate. J Magn Reson Imaging 1994;4:614–6.

6 BONE DEVELOPMENT
AND GROWTH

OSTEOGENESIS

Bone is formed by two methods of differentiation of mesenchymal tissue that may be of either mesodermal or ectomesenchymal (neural crest) origin. The two varieties of ossification are described as intramembranous and endochondral. In both, however, the fundamental laying down of osteoid matrix by osteoblasts and its calcification by amorphous and crystalline apatite deposition are similar.

Intramembranous ossification occurs in sheetlike osteogenic membranes whereas endochondral ossification occurs in hyaline cartilage prototype models of the future bone. The adult structure of osseous tissue formed by the two methods is indistinguishable; furthermore, both methods can participate in forming what may eventually become a single bone, with the distinctions of its different origins effaced. In the main, the long bones of the limbs and the bones of the thoracic cage and cranial base are of endochondral origin whereas those of the vault of the skull, the mandible, and clavicle are predominantly of intramembranous origin. Membrane bones appear to be of neural crest origin, and they arise after the ectomesenchyme interacts with an epithelium.

Control over initiation of osteogenesis resides not in the preosteogenic cells but in adjacent tissues with which they interact inductively. Two genes, core-binding factor alpha 1 (Cbfa-1) and Indian hedgehog (IHH), have been shown to control osteoblast differentiation. Bone morphogenetic proteins (BMPs), members of the transforming growth factor-β (TGF-β) superfamily, and fibroblast growth factors (FGFs) and their receptors (FGFRs) induce bone formation at genetically designated sites (ossification centers). Superimposed on the regulation by transcription and growth factors is the endocrine regulation of osteoblasts and osteoclasts. Differentation of osteoblasts from mesenchyme precedes osteoclast differentiation. Bone deposition by osteoblasts is constantly counterbalanced by osteoclastic bone resorption in a process called bone remodeling, regulated by counteracting hypercalcemic parathyroid hormone and hypocalcemic calcitonin. Superimposed on these two hormones is the control exerted by the sex steroid hormones, particularly estrogens. Delayed onset of osteogenesis will reduce the final size of a bone, and premature onset of osteogenesis will increase its final size. Ontogenetically, such timing variation expresses a person's ultimate size range.

During the 7th week post conception, mesenchymal cells condense as a prelude to both intramembranous and endochondral bone formation. In the former, cells differentiate into osteoblasts that induce osteoid matrix, thereby forming a center of ossification. In the latter, the condensed mesenchymal cells initially form a cartilaginous matrix of glycoproteins; this creates a cartilage model of the future bone. Once it has mineralized, the osteoid matrix forms a collar of periosteal bone surrounding the cartilage. Invasion and replacement of the cartilage model by bone completes endochondral ossification. Growth of endochondral bones depends upon expansion of retained cartilage (epiphyses) and conversion into bone.

Endochondral bone is three-dimensional in its growth pattern, ossifying from one or more deeply seated and slowly expanding centers. The capacity of cartilage for interstitial growth expansion allows for directed prototype cartilage growth; the cartilage "template" is then replaced by endochondral bone, accounting for indirect bone growth. By contrast, intramembranous bone growth is by direct deposition of osseous tissue in osteogenic (periosteal) membranes; this creates accretional growth, often with great speed, especially at fracture sites or over rapidly growing areas such as the frontal lobes of the brain.

Certain inherited congenital defects of bone formation are confined to one type of ossification. Thus, achondroplasia affects only bones of endochondral origin whereas cleidocranial dysostosis afflicts only those bones of intramembranous origin. In contrast, the inherited condition of osteogenesis imperfecta afflicts all bones, whether of endochondral or intramembranous origin.

Ossification starts at definable points in membranes or cartilages; from these centers, ossification radiates into the precursor membrane or cartilage. (An accurate and complete timetable of the onset of prenatal ossification of all bones is still unavailable.) Secondary cartilages that are not part of the cartilaginous primordium of the embryo appear in certain membrane bones (mandible, clavicle) after the onset of intramembranous ossification. Endochondral ossification occurs later in these secondary cartilages of intramembranous bone. The distinction between intramembranous and endochondral bone, although useful at the embryologic level of osteogenesis, tends to become insignificant in postnatal life. For example, during the repair of a fracture to intramembranous bone, cartilage may appear in the healing callus, thereby contradicting its embryologic origins. Further, the subsequent remodeling of initially endochondral bones by surface resorption and deposition by the membranous periosteum or endosteum replaces most endochondral bone with intramembranous bone. Consequently, most endochondral bones become a blend of endochondral and intramembranous components.

In the fetus or newborn, a primary center of ossification first appears; this may be followed by one or more secondary centers, all of which coalesce into a single bone. Most primary ossification centers appear before birth whereas secondary centers appear postnatally. Skeletal growth is interrupted during the neonatal period; this interruption accounts for the natal growth-arrest line in infant bones and teeth. There is evidence of an osteogenesis-inhibiting mechanism in embryonic sutural tissue, accounting for the development of discrete skull bones. Separate bones may fuse into a single composite bone either as a phylogenetic phenomenon, exemplified in the cranial base, or as an ontogenetic phenomenon, exemplified in the fusion of several bones of the skull calvaria into a single bone in extreme old age.

Details of the mechanisms of ossification and the processes of calcification, deposition, and resorption of bone through the operation of osteoblasts and osteoclasts are best studied in histology and physiology texts. The dependence of osseous tissue upon the metabolism of calcium and phosphates means that the structure of bone is a sensitive indicator of the state of turnover of these and other bone minerals. Moreover, bone growth, maintenance, repair, and degeneration depend on the actions of certain hormones and vitamins, which operate indirectly through control of calcium, phosphate, and general metabolism or directly by their varying influences on growth cartilages. An appreciation of these complex physiologic and biochemical phenomena is necessary for understanding the mechanisms of morphogenesis of adult bone structure and shape, but a discussion of this is outside the scope of the present work. (An additional factor of significance in bone physiology and morphology is the hemopoietic function. Bone marrow hemopoiesis begins in the 3rd month post conception and rapidly replaces liver hemopoiesis as the chief site of blood cell formation.)

MORPHOLOGIC DEVELOPMENT

The basic shape and (to a considerable degree) size of bones are genetically determined. Once this inherited morphology is established, environmentally variable minor features of bones (such as ridges, etc.) develop. Superimposed on the basic bone architecture are nutritional, hormonal, and functional influences that, because of the slow and continual replacement of osseous tissue throughout life, enable bones to respond morphologically to functional stresses. Specific periosteal and capsular functional matrices influence specific portions of related bones, termed *skeletal units*. *Macroskeletal units* may consist of a single bone or adjacent portions of several bones (eg, the frontal, parietal, and temporal bones of the calvaria). Each macroskeletal unit is made up of *microskeletal units* that respond independently to functional matrices and thereby determine the varying shapes of the macroskeletal unit or classically named bone. Although the specific growth rates of the individual microskeletal units might differ, there is nonetheless a constant proportionality between growth rates, thereby imparting a fairly constant shape to the enlarging macroskeletal unit.

Based on the influence of muscles on bone morphology, three classes of morphologic features of the craniofacial skeleton have been identified: (1) those that never appear unless muscles are present (eg, temporal line, nuchal lines), (2) those that are self-differentiating but that require muscles to persist (eg, the angular process of mandible), and (3) those that are largely independent of the muscles with which they are associated (eg, the zygomatic bone or the body of the mandible).

The exact mechanism by which functional deforming mechanical forces produce structural bone changes is obscure. One theory postulates mediation of biomechanical stresses through piezoelectric currents created by bioelectric factors. Bone, whose collagen and apatite content renders it highly crystalline, behaves as a crystal when it is mechanically deformed: it generates a minute electric current, thereby producing polar electric fields. Bioelectric effects may be generated in several cell membranes. It is conceivable that osteoclasts and osteoblasts and the matrix within which they operate react to electric potentials by building up bone (experiments suggest) in negatively charged fields and conversely, resorbing bone in positively charged fields. These stress potential currents may allow for the adjustments in bone structure that are made to meet new functional demands.

Another theory of bone remodeling is a mechanochemical hypothesis according to which mechanical stresses are translated into osteoblastic/osteoclastic activity. A change in bone loading results in an altered straining of hydroxyapatite crystals that alters their solubility, changing local calcium activity that either stimulates or resorbs bone.

In orthodontics, a distinction is made between genetically determined unalterable basal bone and the superimposed functional bone that is amenable to manipulated alteration. In practice, "basal" bone refers to the body of the maxilla or mandible, and "functional" bone is the alveolar bone of both jaws that supports the teeth and responds to orthodontic forces. The ultimate shape of a bone and its internal architecture, then, is a reflection of the bone's inherited form and the mechanical demands to which the bone is subjected. Intrinsic genetic factors may play only an initial role in determining the size, shape, and growth of a bone. Extrinsic functional or environmental factors become the predominant determinator of bone form. Because the environment is constantly changing, bones never attain a final morphology, and their shapes are continually subject to change. It has been observed that a bone is composed of the minimal quantity of osseous tissue that will withstand the usual functional stresses applied to it. This supposedly accounts for the hollow marrow centers of long bones and possibly for the sinuses in the skull bones. These factors were formulated into a trajectorial theory of bone structure by Culmann and Meyer just after the middle of the nineteenth century and were proposed as Wolff's law (1870), which states that changes in the function of a bone are attended by alterations in its structure.

GROWTH

During adolescence, there is a bone growth spurt that is believed to be mediated by circulating growth hormones. Bones may differ in the timing of their maximal increases within individuals, suggesting that intrinsic factors in different skull bones may be important in determining changes in the rate of growth at different ages. Circulating growth hormones alone do not determine the timing of the adolescent growth spurt. The pattern of timing of variations in bone growth velocity is intrinsically and (presumably) genetically determined. Hormones augment a genetically regulated pattern of growth rate in the cranial base.

An interposed cartilage (ie, an epiphysis) converting to osseous tissue adds to an endochondral bone's length and simultaneously displaces adjacent parts of the bone by expansion in opposite directions.* Embryonic cartilage cells are

---

*The bones of teleost fishes do not have cartilaginous growth plates. Appositional growth of their bones has no limit. Amphibians and reptiles possess cartilaginous epiphyses that persist throughout life, providing for potentially continuous growth. The osseous fusion of mammalian epiphyses limits the growth potential of their bones.

arranged haphazardly, precluding directionality of growth. By contrast, specialized (epiphyseal) growth plates contain organized columns of cartilage cells, accounting for highly directed growth. This direction-oriented growth is based on chondrocytes being stacked in coinlike columns and on their proliferation acting as hydraulic jacks. Cartilage can grow under weight pressure due to its avascularity; its nutrition is provided by perfusing tissue fluids that are not obstructed by load pressures. For the most part, the growth forces originate within the bone's cartilage. On the other hand, most intramembranous bones with sutural contacts become separated by external capsular functional matrix growth forces (eg, the expanding brain or eyeball). The addition of osseous tissue to these membranous sutural surfaces passively fills in the widened interval in a field of tension, in contrast to the compression field created by the endochondral mechanism.

The overall growth of bones, resulting in their recognizable expansion, is a function of two phenomena: remodeling and transposition. Remodeling is a combination of accretional growth and resorption of bone and is a response, at least in part, to periosteal functional matrices. Because of the rigid nature of calcified bone, growth of this tissue must be appositional by cortical surface deposition of newly formed bone. This primary mode of bone growth contrasts with the interstitial form of growth that takes place in most soft tissues, which can expand by division and growth of cells within the tissue (Fig. 6–1); such internal expansion is not possible in rigid bone. Concomitant with the deposition of bone in certain areas, resorption occurs in other areas to allow for remodeling (ie, changing the shape of a bone). The periosteum covering the surface of bone provides a ready source of osteoblasts for deposition and osteoclasts for resorption. The rate of remodeling diminishes when growth slows down, and bone density increases.

The second basic phenomenon of bone growth, transposition, is the displacement of the remodeling bones vis-à-vis each other. Bone displacement is the result of forces exerted by the surrounding soft tissues (capsular matrices) and by the primary intrinsic growth of the bones themselves. Accordingly, bone growth overall represents the cumulative effects of intrinsic remodeling (a vector of deposition and resorption) and displacement. These phenomena may occur in the same or diverse directions, but their combination is usually

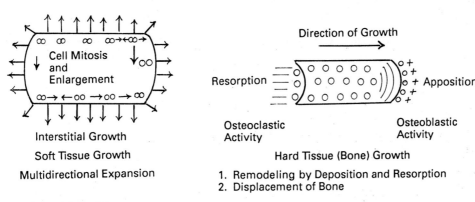

Interstitial Growth

Soft Tissue Growth

Multidirectional Expansion

++ Deposition of Bone

-- Resorption of Bone

Direction of Growth

Resorption — Apposition

Osteoclastic Activity

Osteoblastic Activity

Hard Tissue (Bone) Growth

1. Remodeling by Deposition and Resorption
2. Displacement of Bone

Figure 6–1 Modes of growth.

complex, and their relative contributions are difficult to determine. This difficulty is the source of much controversy relating to craniofacial bone growth.

BONE ARTICULATIONS

Because the sites of junction between bones, known as articulations or joints, are important in relation to bone growth, it is useful to classify them at this juncture. These sites can be classified as movable joints (diarthroses) or immovable joints (synarthroses).

All movable joints are characterized by a synovial membrane lining a joint cavity. Synovial joints are classified according to the shapes of the participating bones (eg, ball-and-socket joints) or the nature of their action (eg, hinge joints).

Diarthroses, per se, do not play a significant role in bone growth except in the case of the temporomandibular joint: the articular cartilage of this joint, alone of all the articular cartilages, provides a growth potential for one of the articulating bones, the mandible.

Synarthroses, on the other hand, play a very significant part in the growth of the articulating bones. Types and examples of immovable joints are shown in Fig. 6–2 and in the following table.

Junctional Tissue	Articulation Type	Example
Fibrous connective tissue	Syndesmosis	Skull suture
Cartilage	Synchondrosis	Symphysis pubis
Bone	Synostosis	Symphysis menti

The apposition of bone during growth may take two forms: (1) surface deposition, accounting for increased thickness of bone that may be modified in remodeling by selective resorption; and (2) sutural deposition, restricted to the opposing edges of bones at a suture site and accounting for the "filling in" of expanded sutures as a result of displacement. Both methods of bone growth are used in different areas of the skull for its expansion in size and its remodeling. Remodeling of growing bone maintains proportions within and between bones. Sutural planes tend to be aligned at right angles to the direction of movement of growing bones. The bony surfaces are oriented to slide in relation to one another as the growing bones move apart. Displacement of bones is an important factor in the expansion of the craniofacial skeleton. The sliding characteristic of bone movement at angled sutural surfaces accommodates the need for continued skeletal growth and determines the direction of growth. The basic suture type is the "butt-end" (or flat end-to-end) type. Beveling and serrations create a second suture type that occurs in sutures in response to functional demands (Fig. 6–3). Sutural serrations are a gross manifestation of a form of trabecular growth responsive to tensions within the sutural tissues, set up in all probability by the rapidly expanding brain, eyeball, nasal septum, etc.

Incremental growth at sutures does not take place only in the plane of the pre-existing curved bones. Differential rates of marginal and surface growth at

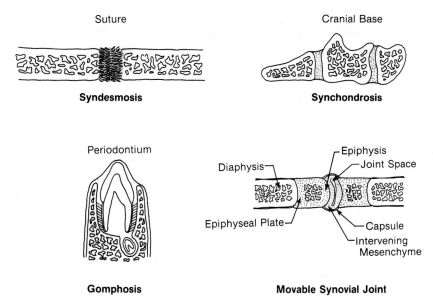

Figure 6–2 Various types of joints.

the suture site allow the plane of growth to alter as the bone edges grow. Resorption of surface bone plays a significant role in this remodeling process. Differential apposition of bone leads to greater or lesser growth of the individual sutural bones, each bony margin contributing independently of the other. In this manner, both remodeling and growth can take place at suture sites. The sutural growth potential is used to advantage in the orthodontic treatment of skeletal deficiencies by techniques of forced expansion, as in the intermaxillary expansion of narrow palates.

Sutural fusion, by ossification of the syndesmotic articulation, indicates cessation of growth at that suture. There is great variability in the timing of sutural closures, making them an unreliable criterion of age. Premature synostosis reduces the cranial diameter at right angles to the fused suture, and abnormal compensatory growth in other directions results in malformation of

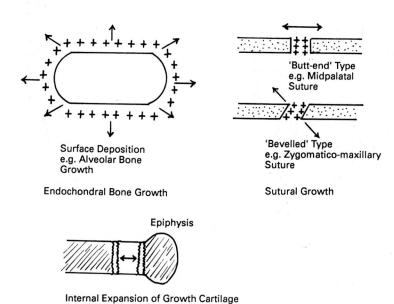

Figure 6–3
Modes of bone growth.

the skull (eg, scaphocephaly [wedge-shaped cranium] and acrocephaly or pla-giocephaly [pointed or twisted cranium]) (see Chapter 14).

Selected Bibliography

Canalis E, editor. Skeletal growth factors. Philadelphia: Lippincott Williams and Wilkins; 2000.

Delezoide AL, Benoist-Lasselin C, Legeai-Mallet L, et al. Spatio-temporal expression of FGFR 1, 2 and 3 genes during human embryo-fetal ossification. Mech Dev 1998;77:19–30.

Ducy P, Zhang R, Geoffroy V, et al. Osf2/Cbfa1: a transcriptional activator of osteoblast differentiation. Cell 1997;89:747–54.

Ducy P, Schinke T, Karsenty G. The osteoblast: a sophisticated fibroblast under central surveillance. Science 2000;289:1501–4.

Goode J, editor. The molecular basis of skeletogenesis. Novartis Foundation vol. 232. Chichester (UK): John Wiley and Sons; 2000.

Hall BK. Bone: a treatise. Vols. I–VII. Boca Raton: CRC Press, Inc.;1991.

Hillarby MC, King KE, Brady G, et al. Localization of gene expression during endo-chondral ossification. Ann N Y Acad Sci 1996;785:263–6.

Karsenty G. The genetic transformation of bone biology. Genes Dev 1999;13:3037–51.

Liu F, Malaval L, Aubin JE. The mature osteoblast phenotype is characterized by extensive plasticity. Exp Cell Res 1997;232:97–105.

O'Rahilly R, Gardner E. The embryology of bone and bones. In: Ackerman LV et al, editors. Bones and joints. Baltimore: Williams and Wilkins; 1976.

Rice D. Molecular mechanisms in calvarial bone and suture development. Dissertationes Biocentri Viikki Universitatis Helsingiensis. Helsinki: Yliopistopaino; 1999.

Teitelbaum SL. Bone resorption by osteoclasts. Science 2000;289:1504–8.

Thorogood P, Sarkar S, Moore R. Skeletogenesis in the head. In: Guggenheim, B, Shapiro, S, editors. Oral biology at the turn of the century. Basel: S. Karger AG; 1998. p. 93–100.

Wezeman FH. Morphological foundations of precartilage development in mesenchyme. Microsc Res Tech 1998;43:91–101.

SECTION II

CRANIOFACIAL DEVELOPMENT

In the closest union there is still some separate existence of component parts; in the most complete separation there is still a reminiscence of union.

Samuel Butler, The Notebooks

INTRODUCTION

The development of the skull (comprising both the cranium and the mandible) is a blend of the morphogenesis and growth of three main skull entities arising from neural crest and paraxial mesoderm tissues. These skull entities are composed of the following:

Embryonic origins of the skull

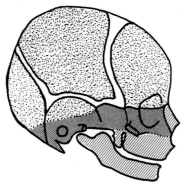

☐ Desmocranium *calvaria- paraxial mesodermal + neural crest*
◼ Chondrocranium
▨ Viscerocranium

Main developmental divisions of the skull

1. The Neurocranium, comprising the following:
   - Vault of the Skull, or Calvaria: phylogenetically of recent origin, to cover the newly expanded brain. The calvaria is formed from intramembranous bone of paraxial mesodermal and neural crest origin; known as the desmocranium (from desmos, membrane)
   - Cranial Base: derived from the phylogenetically ancient cranial floor, associated with the capsular investments of the nasal and auditory sense organs; formed from endochondral bone of neural crest origin; its cartilaginous precursor is known as the chondrocranium (from *chondros*, cartilage)
2. The Face (Orognathofacial Complex): derived from modifications of the phylogenetically ancient branchial-arch structures; formed from intramembranous bone of neural crest origin; also known as the splanchnocranium (from *splanchnos*, viscus) or viscerocranium (from *viscus*, organ), forms the visual, aural, olfactory, and respiratory aditus and the oromasticatory apparatus
3. The Masticatory Apparatus: composed of the jaw bones, their joints and musculature, and the teeth. The dentition is derived phylogenetically from

ectodermal placoid scales, reflected in the embryologic development of the teeth from oral ectoderm (dental lamina) and neural crest (dental papilla)

To some extent, the cranial base is shared by both neurocranial and facial elements. The masticatory apparatus is composed of both facial and dental elements. The skull is thus a mosaic of individual components, each of which grows to the proper extent and in the proper direction to attain and maintain the stability of the whole.

Each of the three main craniofacial entities possesses different characteristics of growth, development, maturation, and function, yet each unit is so integrated with the others that coordination of the growth of all is required for normal development. Failure of correlation of the differing growth patterns or aberration of inception or growth of an individual component results in distorted craniofacial relationships and is a factor in the development of dental malocclusion. Although both the neurocranium and the face have mixed intramembranous and endochondral types of bone formation, the bony elements of the masticatory apparatus are predominantly of intramembranous origin. The dental tissues have an ectodermal origin for their enamel and a neural crest origin for much of the mesenchyme that forms the dentine, pulp, cementum, and periodontal ligament.

Interestingly, the historically more recent developments in the mammalian skull (ie, the membrane bones of the jaws and facial skeleton [splanchnocranium]) are more susceptible to developmental anomalies than are the older cartilaginous parts of the skull (the chondrocranium). Developmental defects of the face and jaws are relatively common whereas congenital defects of the skull base and the nasal and otic (auditory) capsules are relatively rare. During the postnatal growth of congenital craniofacial defects, three general patterns of development have been observed. In the first, hypoplastic defects may improve, with "catch-up" growth minimizing the defect. In the second, the defective pattern of growth is maintained throughout infancy or childhood, so that the malformation is retained to the same degree in the adult. In the third pattern, the developmental derangement worsens with age, the severity of the malformation becoming greater in adulthood.

Differentiation and growth of the chondrocranium appear to be strongly genetically determined and subject to minimal environmental influence. Diseases of defective endochondral bone formation are reflected in abnormalities of the skull base. On the other hand, growth of the desmocranium and splanchnocranium appears to be subject to minimal genetic determination but strongly influenced by local environmental factors.

The cranial components surrounding the sense organs of olfaction, sight, hearing, and balance are almost fully grown at birth. The remaining cranial elements grow and change considerably postnatally, in keeping with the enlargement and use of adjacent structures. The calvaria grows most rapidly in response to the early expanding brain, followed by the nasal airway system determining midfacial development. The masticatory system is the last major functional system to reach maturity.

For descriptive convenience, details of the growth and development of the head have been subdivided into the following components:

- The calvaria
- The cranial base
- The facial skeleton
- The palate
- The paranasal sinuses
- The mandible
- The temporomandibular joint
- Skull growth: sutures and cephalometrics
- The tongue and tonsils
- The salivary glands
- Muscle development
- The special-sense organs
- The dentition

7 CALVARIA AND THE MEMBRANOUS NEUROCRANIUM (DESMOCRANIUM)

NORMAL DEVELOPMENT

The mesenchyme that gives rise to the vault of the neurocranium is arranged first as a capsular membrane around the developing brain. The membrane is composed of two layers: (1) an inner *endomeninx*, primarily of neural crest origin, and (2) an outer *ectomeninx*, of mixed paraxial mesodermal and neural crest origin (Fig. 7–1). The endomeninx forms the two leptomeningeal coverings of the brain—the pia mater and the arachnoid. The ectomeninx dif-

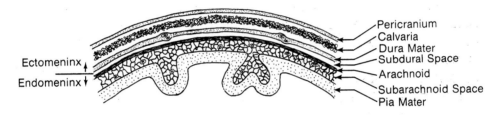

Figure 7–1 Neurocranial derivatives of the embryonic ectomeninx (calvaria and dura mater) and endomeninx (arachnoid and pia mater).

ferentiates into the inner dura mater, which covers the brain and remains unossified, and an outer superficial membrane with chondrogenic and osteogenic properties. Osteogenesis of the ectomeninx occurs as intramembranous bone formation over the expanding dome of the brain, forming the skull vault or calvaria, whereas the ectomeninx forming the floor of the brain chondrifies as the chondrocranium, which later ossifies endochondrally (Fig. 7–2).

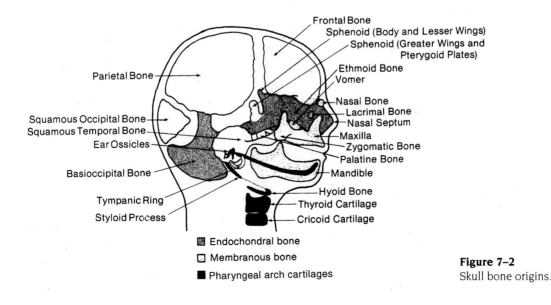

Figure 7–2
Skull bone origins.

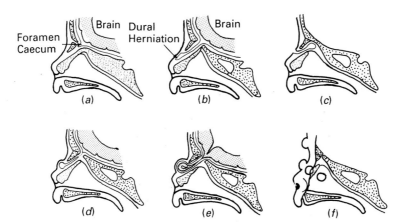

Figure 7–3 Patterns of meningoencephalocele herniation through the foramen caecum, forming facial defects. (*a*) Embryonic stage; the dura is within the foramen caecum. (*b*) During fetal development, the dura herniates through the foramen caecum and contacts skin; it normally retracts before birth. (*c*) Dermoid sinus with cyst. (*d*) Dermoid cyst, which may or may not have a stalk to the dura. (*e*) Encephalocele. (*f*) Possible sites of defects.

Despite their divergent fates, the two layers of the ectomeninx remain in close apposition except in regions where the venous sinuses develop. The dura mater and its septa (the falces cerebri and cerebelli and the tentorium cerebelli) show distinctly organized fiber bundles closely related and strongly attached to the sutural systems that later develop in the vault. The adult form of the neurocranium is the end result of the preferential direction of the forces set up by growth of the brain constrained by these dural fiber systems. Without the dural bands, the brain would expand as a perfect sphere. Because the dura mater serves as the endocranial periosteum, it also determines the shape of the calvarial bones.

In the somite period embryo, the neural tube's covering dura mater and its surface ectoderm are in contact in the area of the closing anterior neuropore of the developing brain. Transient maintenance of this contact during development causes a dural projection that, because of the ventral bending of the rostrum, extends into the future frontonasal suture area. Later, as the nasal capsules surround the dural projection, the resulting midline canal forms the basis of the foramen caecum where the ethmoid-frontal bone junction develops. The dural projection and frontonasal area skin normally separate, allowing the canal to close, forming the foramen caecum (hence its name, meaning "blind foramen"). If the foramen fails to close, an abnormal pathway for neural tissue to herniate into the nasal region results. Herniated portions of the brain are known as *encephaloceles*, congenital anomalies most commonly seen in the frontal bone and occipital regions (Fig. 7–3).

Ossification of the intramembranous calvarial bones depends on the presence of the brain; in its absence (anencephaly), no bony calvaria forms (see Fig. 3–19 in Chapter 3). Several primary and secondary ossification centers develop in the outer layer of the ectomeninx, to form individual bones. The mesodermally derived ectomeninx gives rise to major portions of the frontal, parietal, sphenoid, petrous temporal, and occipital bones (Fig. 7–4). The neural crest provides the mesenchyme forming the lacrimal, nasal, squamous

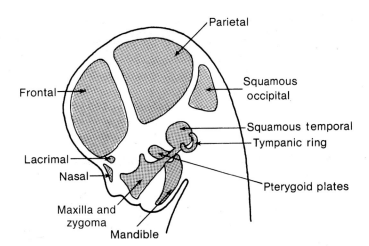

Figure 7–4 Ossification sites of membranous skull bones.

temporal, zygomatic, maxillary, and mandibular bones. These embryonic distinctions of bone derivation account for different syndromic characteristics of bone lesions in neurocristopathies versus mesodermal-based pathologic lesions.

A pair of frontal bones appears from single primary ossification centers, forming in the region of each superciliary arch at the 8th week post conception. Three pairs of secondary centers appear later in the zygomatic processes, nasal spine, and trochlear fossae. Fusion between these centers is complete at 6 to 7 months post conception. At birth, the frontal bones are separated by the frontal (metopic) suture; synostotic fusion of this suture usually starts about the 2nd year and unites the frontal bones into a single bone by 7 years of age. (The frontal [metopic] suture persists into adulthood in 10 to 15% of skulls. In such cases, the frontal sinuses are absent or hypoplastic.)

The two parietal bones arise from two primary ossification centers for each bone that appear at the parietal eminence in the 8th week post conception and fuse in the 4th month post conception. Delayed ossification in the region of the parietal foramina may result in a sagittal fontanelle at birth.

The supranuchal squamous portion of the occipital bone (above the superior nuchal line) ossifies intramembranously from two centers, one on each side, appearing in the 8th week post conception. The rest of the occipital bone ossifies endochondrally (see p. 93).

The squamous portion of the temporal bone* ossifies intramembranously from a single center appearing at the root of the zygoma at the 8th week post conception. The tympanic ring of the temporal bone ossifies intramembranously from four centers, appearing in the lateral wall of the tympanum in the 3rd month after conception. The two membranous bone portions of the temporal bone fuse at birth. The rest of the temporal bone ossifies endochondrally (see p. 94).

Should any unusual ossification centers develop between individual calvarial bones, their independent existence is recognizable as small sutural or

---

*The squamous temporal bone is independent of brain induction and is present in anencephaly.

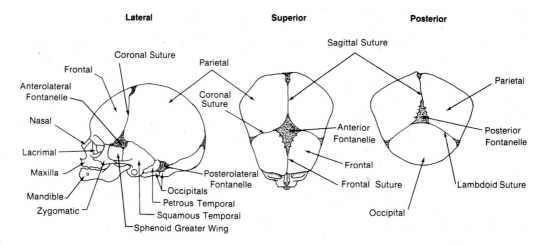

Figure 7–5 Fontanelles and sutures of the calvaria.

wormian bones.* The earliest centers of ossification first appear during the 7th and 8th weeks post conception, but ossification is not completed until well after birth. The mesenchyme between the bones develops fibers to form syndesmotic articulations. The membranous mesenchyme covering the bones forms the periosteum. At birth, the individual calvarial bones are separated by sutures of variable width and by fontanelles. Six of these fontanelles are identified as the anterior, posterior, posterolateral, and anterolateral fontanelles, in relation to the corners of the two parietal bones (Fig. 7–5). These flexible membranous junctions between the calvarial bones allow the narrowing of the sutures and fontanelles and the overriding of these bones when they become compressed in traversing the pelvic birth canal during birth. The head may appear distorted for several days after birth (Fig. 7–6).

Postnatal bone growth results in narrowing of the sutures and elimination of the fontanelles. The anterolateral fontanelles close 3 months after birth; the posterolateral ones close during the 2nd year. (The site of the anterolateral

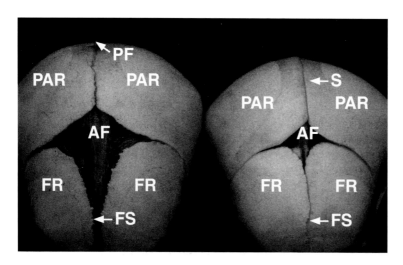

Figure 7–6 Top view of the calvariae of two neonate skulls, depicting the variability of anterior fontanelle size at birth. AF, anterior fontanelle; FR, frontal bone; FS, frontal (metopic) suture; PAR, parietal bone; PF, posterior fontanelle; S, sagittal suture.

*Wormian bones occur most frequently along the lambdoid suture, where they form interparietal bones. Development of these ossicles may have a genetic component; but as nearly all hydrocephalic crania have wormian bones, it appears that deforming stress is a contributing factor.

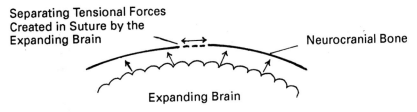

Figure 7–7 Schematic section through skull and brain to demonstrate the forces of "functional matrix" growth.

fontanelle corresponds to pterion in the adult skull; the site of the posterolateral fontanelle corresponds to asterion.) The posterior fontanelle closes 2 months after birth, and the anterior one closes during the 2nd year. The median frontal suture is usually obliterated between 6 and 8 years of age. Fusion of the frontal (metopic) suture involves chondroid tissue, occasionally forming secondary cartilage, which is progressively substituted by lamellar bone. This extended ossification of the calvarial bones continues throughout life: the syndesmosal sutures between the neurocranial bones fuse into synostoses with advancing years, uniting the individual calvarial bones into a single component in old age. In the fetus, the intramembranous neurocranial bones are molded into large, slightly curved "plates" over the expanding brain that they cover.

The precocious development of the brain determines the early predominance of the neurocranium over the facial and masticatory portions of the skull. Although the brain and (consequently) the neurocranial bone vault develop very rapidly very early, their growth slows and ceases at an earlier age than the growth of the facial and masticatory elements of the skull. The predominance of the neurocranium over the face is greatest in the early fetus, reducing to an 8:1 proportion at birth, to 6:1 in the 2nd year, to 4:1 in the 5th year, and from 2:1 to 2.5:1 in the adult. At birth, the neurocranium has achieved 25 percent of its ultimate growth; it completes 50 percent by the age of 6 months and 75 percent by 2 years. By 10 years of age, neurocranial growth is 95 percent complete, but the facial skeleton has achieved only 65 percent of its total growth. In postnatal life, the neurocranium increases 4 to 5 times in volume whereas the facial portion increases some 8 to 10 times its volume at birth.

The ultimate shape and size of the cranial vault primarily depend on the internal pressures exerted on the inner table of the neurocranial bones. The expanding brain exerts separating tensional forces upon the bone sutures, thereby secondarily stimulating compensatory sutural bone growth (Fig. 7–7). The brain acts in this context as a "functional matrix" in determining the extent of neurocranial bone growth. Because it is related to intracranial volume, the circumference of the head is a good indicator of brain growth.* The precocious early development of the brain is reflected in the rapidly enlarging circumference of the head, which nearly doubles from an average of 18 cm at the midges-

---

*Between birth and adulthood, brain size increases about 3½ times, from approximately 400 cm³ to 1,300 to 1,400 cm³. The early rapid expansion of the brain poses problems for the already established cerebral blood vessels; it stretches them, weakening their walls and predisposing them to aneurysm formation in later life.

tational period (4 to 5 months) to an average of 33 cm (approximately 13 in) at birth. This rapid increase of head circumference continues during the 1st year, reaching an average of 46 cm, and then slows; head circumference reaches 49 cm at 2 years and only 50 cm at 3 years. The increase between the age of 3 years and adulthood is only about 6 cm.

Growth of the calvarial bones is a combination of (1) sutural growth, (2) surface apposition and resorption (remodeling), and (3) centrifugal displacement by the expanding brain. The proportions attributable to the various growth mechanisms vary. Accretion to the calvarial bones is predominantly sutural until about the 4th year of life, after which surface apposition becomes increasingly important. Remodeling of the curved bony plates allows for their flattening out to accommodate the increasing surface area of the growing brain. The flattening of the early high curvature of the calvarial bones is achieved by a combination of endocranial erosion and ectocranial deposition, together with ectocranial resorption from certain areas of maximal curvature such as the frontal and parietal eminences.

The bones of the newborn calvaria are unilaminar and lack diploë. From about 4 years of age, lamellar compaction of cancellous trabeculae forms the inner and outer tables of the cranial bones. The tables become continuously more distinct into adulthood. This differential bone structure creates a high stiffness - to - weight ratio, with no relative increase in the mineral content of cranial bone from birth to adulthood. Whereas the behavior of the inner table is related primarily to the brain and intracranial pressures, the outer table is more responsive to extracranial muscular and buttressing forces. However, the two cortical plates are not completely independent. The thickening of the frontal bone in the midline at the glabella results from separation of the inner and outer tables with invasion of the frontal sinus between the cortical plates. Only the external plate is remodeled, as the internal plate becomes stable at 6 to 7 years of age, reflecting the near cessation of cerebral growth. Thus, only the inner aspect of the frontal bone can be used as a stable (x-ray) reference point for growth studies from the age of 7 years onward. Growth of the external plate during childhood produces the superciliary arches, the mastoid processes, the external occipital protuberance, and the temporal and nuchal lines that are all absent from the neonatal skull. The bones of the calvaria continue to thicken slowly even after their general growth is complete.

When intracranial pressures become excessive, as in hydrocephalus, both plates of the bones of the calvaria become thinned and grossly expanded. Conversely, the reduced functional matrix force of the brain in microcephalics results in a small calvaria. Normal forces acting on the outer table of bone alone tend to influence the superstructure of the cranium only, not the intracranial form. To some degree, the pull of muscles would account for the development of the mastoid process, the lateral pterygoid plate, the temporal and nuchal lines in the cranium, the coronoid process, and the ramus-body angle of the mandible. In the face, the buttressing resistance to masticatory forces produces the supraorbital processes, superstructural bony projections that add to the dimension of the cranium but that are unrelated to the intracranial capacity. Abnormal external forces during development can distort cranial mor-

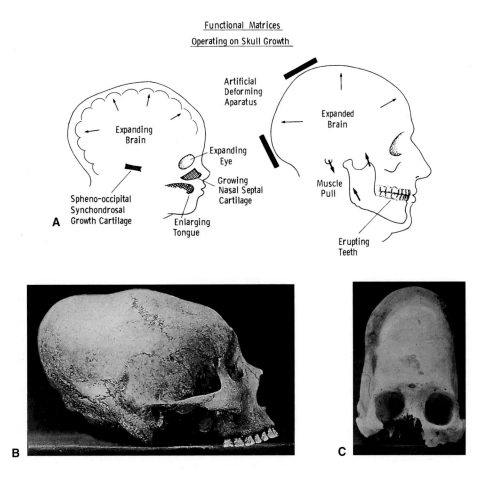

Figure 7–8 (A) Functional matrices operating on skull growth. (B) An adult skull distorted into an anteroposterior elongation by constraining head-boards in infancy. (C) An adult skull distorted into an acrocephalic shape by contraints applied in infancy.

phology but, strangely enough, not cranial capacity, as is evident by the bizarre shapes of skulls produced by pressure devices on children's skulls in some tribal societies. These artificially shaped skulls are named according to their distortions (eg, acrocephaly, platycephaly, brachycephaly, etc.) (Fig. 7–8).

ANOMALIES OF DEVELOPMENT

The calvaria is particularly susceptible to a number of congenital defects ranging from chromosomal to hormonal in their etiology. The time of closure of the sutures is altered in many of these afflictions, leading to variable distortions of skull shape. In such widely different conditions as cretinism, progeria, trisomy 21, and cleidocranial dysostosis, there is delayed midline ossification of the frontal (metopic) and sagittal sutures of the calvaria, so that the anterior fontanelle (the "soft spot" on an infant's head) may remain open into adult life. The resulting brachycephalic skull results in a "bossed" forehead of highly curved frontal and parietal bones and in hypertelorism, partly obscuring the smaller brain case.

Premature fusion of sutures (craniosynostosis) is dealt with in Chapter 14 (p. 148). Defects in closure of the foramen caecum at the ethmoid-frontal suture allow herniation of the cranial contents into the face, forming frontal encephaloceles (see Fig. 7–3). Occipital encephaloceles may occur through cranioschisis (fissured cranium) lesions. Basal encephaloceles protrude through the skull base.

Selected Bibliography

Harris CP, Townsend JJ, Carey JC. Acalvaria: a unique congenital anomaly. Am J Med Genet 1993;46:694–9.

Iseki S, Wilkie AO, Heath JK, et al. Fgfr2 and osteopontin domains in the developing skull vault are mutually exclusive and can be altered by locally applied FGF2. Development 1997;124:3375–84.

Kim HJ, Rice DP, Kettunen PJ, Thesleff I. FGF-, BMP- and Shh-mediated signalling pathways in the regulation of cranial suture morphogenesis and calvarial bone development. Development 1998;125:1241–51.

Liu YH, Kundu R, Wu L, et al. Premature suture closure and ectopic cranial bone in mice expressing Msx2 transgenes in the developing skull. Proc Natl Acad Sci U S A 1995;92:6137–41.

Mandarim-de-Lacerda CA, Alves MU. Growth of the cranial bones in human fetuses (2nd and 3rd trimesters). Surg Radiol Anat 1992;14:125–9.

Neumann K, Moegelin A, Temminghoff M, et al. 3D-computed tomography: a new method for the evaluation of fetal cranial morphology. J Craniofac Genet Dev Biol; 1997;17:9–22.

Silau AM, Fischer Hansen B, Kjaer I. Normal prenatal development of the human parietal bone and interparietal suture. J Craniofac Genet Dev Biol 1995;15:81–6.

Toma CD, Schaffer JL, Meazzini MC, et al. Developmental restriction of embryonic calvarial cell populations as characterized by their in vitro potential for chondrogenic differentiation. J Bone Miner Res 1997;12:2024–39.

Villanueva JE, Nimni ME. Modulation of osteogenesis by isolated calvaria cells: a model for tissue interactions. Biomaterials 1990;11:19–21.

8 CRANIAL BASE

THE CHONDROCRANIUM

During the 4th week post conception, mesenchyme derived from the paraxial mesoderm and neural crest condenses between the developing brain and foregut to form the base of the ectomeningeal capsule. This condensation betokens the earliest evidence of skull formation. Even then, development of the skull starts comparatively late, after the development of the primordia of many of the other cranial structures such as the brain, cranial nerves, eyes, and blood vessels. During the late somite period, the occipital sclerotomal mesenchyme concentrates around the notochord underlying the developing hindbrain. From this region, the mesenchymal concentration extends cephalically, forming a floor for the brain. Conversion of the ectomeninx mesenchyme into cartilage constitutes the beginning of the chondrocranium, starting on the 40th day after conception. Formation of the cartilages of the chondrocranium is dependent on the presence of the brain and other neural structures and on an appropriately staged inducing epithelium. Chondrogenesis will occur only after an epithelial mesenchymal interaction has taken place.

Chondrification centers forming around the cranial end of the notochord are appropriately called the parachordal cartilages (Fig. 8–1). From these, a caudal extension of chondrification incorporates the fused sclerotomes arising from the four occipital somites surrounding the neural tube. The sclerotome cartilage, the first part of the skull to develop, forms the boundaries of the foramen magnum, providing the anlagen for the basilar and condylar parts of the occipital bone.

The cranial end of the notochord is at the level of the oropharyngeal membrane, which closes off the stomodeum. Just cranial to this membrane, the

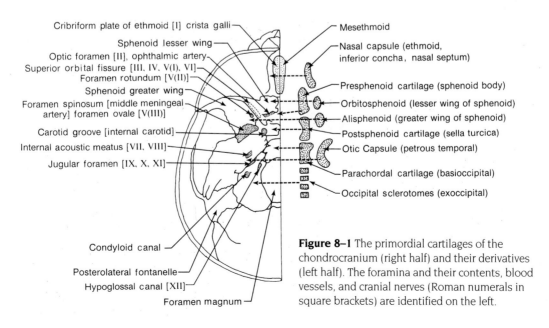

Cribriform plate of ethmoid [I] crista galli
Sphenoid lesser wing
Optic foramen [II], ophthalmic artery
Superior orbital fissure [III, IV, V(I), VI]
Foramen rotundum [V(II)]
Sphenoid greater wing
Foramen spinosum [middle meningeal artery] foramen ovale [V(III)]
Carotid groove [internal carotid]
Internal acoustic meatus [VII, VIII]
Jugular foramen [IX, X, XI]

Mesethmoid
Nasal capsule (ethmoid, inferior concha, nasal septum)
Presphenoid cartilage (sphenoid body)
Orbitosphenoid (lesser wing of sphenoid)
Alisphenoid (greater wing of sphenoid)
Postsphenoid cartilage (sella turcica)
Otic Capsule (petrous temporal)
Parachordal cartilage (basioccipital)
Occipital sclerotomes (exoccipital)

Condyloid canal
Posterolateral fontanelle
Hypoglossal canal [XII]
Foramen magnum

Figure 8–1 The primordial cartilages of the chondrocranium (right half) and their derivatives (left half). The foramina and their contents, blood vessels, and cranial nerves (Roman numerals in square brackets) are identified on the left.

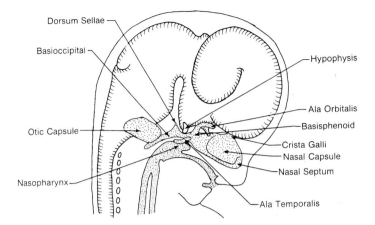

Figure 8–2 Schematic parasagittal section through the head of an early fetus (8th week). The chondrocranium cartilages are identified by wide-spaced stippling.

adenohypophysial (Rathke's) pouch arises from the stomodeum; the pouch gives rise to the anterior lobe of the pituitary gland (adenohypophysis), lying immediately cranial to the termination of the notochord (Fig. 8–2; see also Fig. 3–1 in Chapter 3). Two hypophysial (postsphenoid) cartilages develop on either side of the hypophysial stem and fuse to form the basisphenoid (postsphenoid) cartilage, which contains the hypophysis and which will later give rise to the sella turcica and posterior part of the body of the sphenoid bone.

Cranial to the pituitary gland, fusion of two presphenoid (trabecular) cartilages forms the precursor to the presphenoid bone that will form the anterior part of the body of the sphenoid bone. Laterally, the chondrification centers of the orbitosphenoid (lesser wing) and alisphenoid (greater wing) contribute wings to the sphenoid bone. Most anteriorly, the fused presphenoid cartilages become a vertical cartilaginous plate (the mesethmoid cartilage) within the nasal septum. The mesethmoid cartilage ossifies at birth into the perpendicular plate of the ethmoid bone, its upper edge forming the crista galli that separates the olfactory bulbs (Fig. 8–3).

The capsules surrounding the nasal (olfactory) and otic (vestibulocochlear) sense organs chondrify and fuse to the cartilages of the cranial base. The nasal capsule (ectethmoid)* chondrifies in the 2nd month post conception to form a box of cartilage with a roof and lateral walls divided by a median cartilage sep-

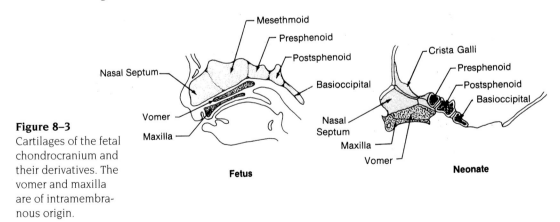

Figure 8–3 Cartilages of the fetal chondrocranium and their derivatives. The vomer and maxilla are of intramembranous origin.

*The nasal capsule and nasal septum have been postulated to arise from prechordal (preotic) sclerotomes; the myotomes of these prechordal somitomeres give rise to the extrinsic eye muscles.

Figure 8–4 Schema of coronal section of nasal capsules and ossification centers.

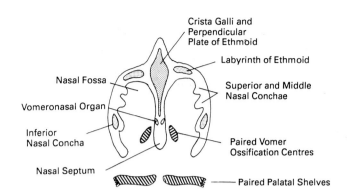

tum (mesethmoid) (Fig. 8–4). Ossification centers in the lateral walls form the lateral masses (labyrinths) of the ethmoid bone and the inferior nasal concha bones.

The median nasal septum remains cartilaginous except posteroinferiorly. There, in the membrane on each side of the septum, intramembranous ossification centers form the initially paired vomer bone, its two halves uniting from below before birth but containing intervening nasal septal cartilage until puberty. The vomerine alae extend posteriorly over the basisphenoid, forming the roof of the nasopharynx—a distinctively human feature. Appositional bone growth postnatally on the posterosuperior margins of the vomer contributes to nasal septal growth and indirectly contributes to the downward and forward growth of the face.

The chondrified nasal capsules form the cartilages of the nostrils and the nasal septal cartilage. In the fetus, the septal cartilage intervenes between the cranial base above and the "premaxilla," vomer, and palatal processes of the maxilla below.* The growth of the nasal septal cartilage is equivocally believed to play a role in the downward and forward growth of the midface (acting as a "functional matrix") (see p. 106).

The otic capsules chondrify and fuse with the parachordal cartilages to ossify later as the mastoid and petrous portions of the temporal bones. The optic capsule does not chondrify in humans.

The initially separate centers of cranial base chondrification fuse into a single, irregular, and much-perforated basal plate. The early (prechondrification) establishment of the blood vessels, cranial nerves, and spinal cord between the developing brain and its extracranial contacts is responsible for the numerous perforations (foramina) in the cartilage basal plate and the subsequent osseous cranial floor (see Fig. 8–1).

The ossifying chondrocranium meets the ossifying desmocranium to form the neurocranium. The developing brain lies in the shallow groove formed by the chondrocranium. The deep central hypophysial fossa is bounded by the presphenoid cartilage of the tuberculum sellae anteriorly and the postsphenoid cartilage of the dorsum sellae posteriorly.

The fibers of the olfactory nerve (I) determine the perforations of the cribriform plate of the ethmoid bone. Extensions of the orbitosphenoid cartilage

---

* Postnatally, the septal cartilage may act as a strut to resist the compressive forces of incision, transferring these forces from the incisor region to the sphenoid bone.

TABLE 8-1 Basicranial Ossification Centers

Bone	Site and Number of Ossification Centers		Initial appearance (weeks)
	Intramembranous	*Endochondral*	
Occipital	Supranuchal squamous (2)	—	8
		Infranuchal squamous (2)	10
		Basilar (1)	11
		Exoccipital (2)	12
Temporal	Squamous (1)	—	8
	Tympanic ring (4)	—	12
	—	Petrosal (14)	16
	—	Styloid (2)	Perinatal
Ethmoid	—	Lateral labyrinths (2)	16
	—	Perpendicular plate; crista (1)	36
Vomer	Alae (2)	—	8
Sphenoid	—	Presphenoid (3)	16
	—	Postsphenoid (4)	16
	—	Orbitosphenoids (2)	9
	—	Alisphenoids (2)	8
	—	Pterygoid hamuli (2)	12
	Medial pterygoid plates (2)	—	8
	Lateral pterygoid plates (2)	—	8
	—	Sphenoidal conchae (2)	20
Inferior nasal concha	—	Lamina (1)	20

around the optic nerve (II) and ophthalmic artery, when fused with the cranial part of the basal plate, form the optic foramen. The space between the orbitosphenoid and alisphenoid cartilages is retained as the superior orbital fissure, a pathway for the oculomotor (III), trochlear (IV), ophthalmic (V1), and abducens (VI) nerves and the ophthalmic veins. The junction of the alisphenoid (greater wing) and presphenoid cartilages of the sphenoid bone is interrupted by pathways of the maxillary nerve (V2), to create the foramen rotundum, and of the mandibular nerve (V3) to create the foramen ovale. The

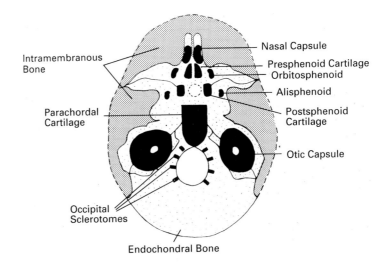

Figure 8–5 Schema of an adult cranial base, indicating sites of primordial cartilages of chondrocranium (in black) and extent of endochondral (light stipple) and intramembranous (heavy stipple) ossification.

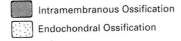

middle meningeal artery forms the foramen spinosum. The persistence of the cartilage between the ossification sites of the alisphenoid and the otic capsule accounts for the foramen lacerum.

Ossification around the internal carotid artery accounts for its canal, interposed at the junction of the alisphenoid and postsphenoid cartilages and otic capsule. The passage of the facial (VII) and vestibulocochlear (VIII) nerves through the otic capsule ensures patency of the internal acoustic meatus. The glossopharyngeal (IX), vagus (X), and spinal accessory (XI) nerves and the internal jugular vein passing between the otic capsule and the parachordal cartilage account for the large jugular foramen. The hypoglossal nerve (XII) passing between the occipital sclerotomes accounts for the hypoglossal or anterior condylar canal. The spinal cord determines the foramen magnum (see Fig. 8–1).

Approximately 110 ossification centers appear in the embryonic human skull (Table 8–1). Many of these centers fuse to produce 45 bones in the neonatal skull. In the young adult, 22 skull bones are recognized.

Centers of ossification within the basal plate, commencing with the alisphenoids in the 8th week post conception, lay the basis for the endochondral bone portions of the occipital, sphenoid, and temporal bones (all of which also have intramembranous bone components) and for the wholly endochondral ethmoid and inferior nasal concha bones (Fig. 8–5).

Unossified chondrocranial remnants persist at birth as the alae and septum of the nose, as the spheno-occipital and sphenopetrous junctions, in the apex of the petrous bone, between the separate parts of the occipital bone, and in the foramen lacerum.

The Occipital Bone

Derived from both the basicranial cartilage (contributed by the occipital sclerotomes) and the desmocranial membrane, the occipital bone ossifies from seven centers (two intramembranous, five endochondral) around the medulla oblongata, which determines the foramen magnum (Fig. 8–6; see also

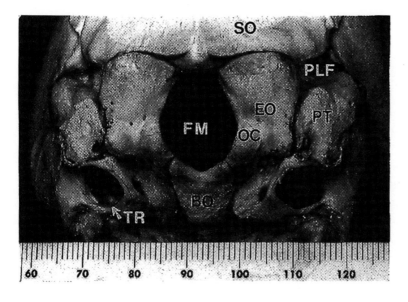

Figure 8–6 Base of a neonatal skull with forming occipital bone surrounding the foramen magnum. Note the synchondroses in the occipital condyles between the exoccipital and basioccipital and the absence of the mastoid processes. BO, basioccipital; EO, exoccipital; FM, foramen magnum; OC occipital condyle; PLF, posterolateral fontanelle; PT, petrous temporal; SO, squamous occipital; TR, tympanic ring.

Fig. 8–5). The occipital bone develops in a modified vertebral pattern, with components representing the centrum, transverse processes, and neural arches of several successive occipital vertebrae. The basioccipital cartilage, like the vertebral bodies, is traversed by the notochord, vestiges of which persist until birth. The squamous portion above the superior nuchal line ossifies from a pair of intramembranous ossification centers in the 8th week post conception, and from a pair of endochondral ossification centers infranuchally in the 10th week. The paired infranuchal chondral segments fuse, and a median wedge of cartilage (Kerckring's center) usually develops posterior to the foramen magnum, but the median intramembranous suture remains unfused at its dorsal margin. The transverse nuchal suture between the cartilaginous and membranous portions of the occipital squama may persist, but it normally fuses by the 12th week in most cases.

The single median basicranial endochondral ossification center appearing at the 11th week forms the basioccipital bone anterior to the foramen magnum and the anterior one-third of the occipital condyles. A pair of endochondral ossification centers appearing at the 12th week form the exoccipital bones, lateral to the foramen magnum, including the posterior two-thirds of the occipital condyles; these surround the hypoglossal nerves to form the hypoglossal canals. The occipital squama starts to fuse with the exoccipitals at the posterior intraoccipital synchondroses during the 2nd or 3rd year postnatally. The exoccipitals join the basioccipital at the anterior intraoccipital synchrondroses, which lie within the condyles. During the 3rd or 4th year, these anterior synchondroses start to disappear; by the age of 7 years, the squamous, exoccipital, and basilar portions have united into a single occipital bone. A pharyngeal tubercle appears on the ventral aspect of the basioccipital to provide attachment for the median pharyngeal raphe. The nuchal lines and the occipital protuberance enlarge postnatally with nuchal muscular usage.

Postnatally, the endocranial surfaces of the occipital bone are predominantly resorptive, and the ectocranial surfaces are depositary, resulting in the downward displacement of the floor of the posterior cranial fossa to accommodate the enlarging brain. The squamous and basilar portions have independent rates of growth.

The Temporal Bone

The squamous and tympanic components of the temporal bone ossify intramembranously whereas the petrosal and styloid elements ossify endochondrally from some 21 ossification centers. The squamous portion ossifies intramembranously from a single center appearing in the 8th week post conception; the zygomatic process extends from this ossification center. The tympanic ring surrounding the external acoustic meatus ossifies from four intramembranous centers, starting in the 3rd month post conception. The inner-ear otocyst induces chondrogenesis in the periotic mesenchyme, of both neural crest and mesodermal origin, to form the otic capsule; local repression of chondrogenesis accounts for the perilymphatic space within the capsule. The petrosal part ossifies endochondrally in the otic capsule from about 14 centers; the centers first appear in the 16th week around the nerves of the inner ear and fuse during the 6th month post conception, when the contained inner-ear labyrinth has reached its final size. The otic capsule is initially continuous with the basioccipital cartilage, but the synchondrosis converts to the foramen lacerum and jugular foramen.

The middle ear within the petrosal bone contains derivatives of the first and second pharyngeal arches that form the malleus, incus, and stapes bones (see p. 54).

The petrosal bone forming the adult otic capsule consists of three layers. The inner endosteal and outer periosteal layers contain haversian canals whereas the middle layer consists of highly mineralized endochondral fetal-type bone that (uniquely) is retained throughout life and is not replaced by canalicular haversian bone. The osseous labyrinth, as an inner woven bone capsule protecting the membranous labyrinth, remains unaltered throughout life. By contrast, the petrosal outer periosteal layer remodels to lamellar bone and adapts to functional stresses. The styloid process ossifies from two centers in the hyoid (second) pharyngeal-arch cartilage (see p. 55); the upper center appears just before birth, and the lower center appears just after birth.

At 22 weeks after conception, the petrous part and tympanic ring fuse incompletely, leaving the petrotympanic fissure through which the chorda tympani nerve and remnants of the diskomalleolar ligament pass. At birth, the tympanic ring fuses incompletely with the squamous part of the temporal bone, forming the persisting squamotympanic fissure. Later, the ring grows laterally to form the tympanic plate. The petrous, squamous, and proximal styloid process portions fuse during the 1st year of life, and the distal and proximal styloid processes fuse at about puberty.

The mandibular (glenoid) fossa is only a shallow depression at birth, deepening with the development of the articular eminence (see Chapter 13). The mastoid process develops after the 2nd year, when it is invaded by extensions of the tympanic antrum to form mastoid air cells.

The Ethmoid Bone

The wholly endochondral ethmoid bone, which forms the median floor of the anterior cranial fossa and parts of the roof, lateral walls, and median septum of the nasal cavity, ossifies from three centers. A single median center in the mesethmoid cartilage forms the perpendicular plate and crista galli just before birth; a pair of centers for the lateral labyrinths appears in the nasal capsular cartilages at the 4th month post conception; and a secondary ossification center appears between the cribriform plates and crista galli at birth (see Fig. 8–4). At 2 years of age, the perpendicular plate unites with the labyrinths, through fusion of the cribriform plate, to form a single ethmoid bone.

Resorption of the endocranial surface of the cribriform plates, with deposition on the opposite nasal surface, results in the downward movement of the anterior cranial floor. Postnatal growth of the cribriform plate is slight and is complete by 4 years of age. Postnatal growth of the other nasal elements is a potent factor in the enlargement of the middle third of the face.

The Inferior Nasal Concha

An endochondral bone, the inferior nasal concha ossifies in the cartilage of the lateral part of the nasal capsule (the ectethmoid) from a single center that appears in the 5th month post conception (see Fig. 8–4). Peripheral ossification of the cartilaginous scroll creates a double bony lamella when the cartilage resorbs. The inferior concha detaches from the ectethmoid to become an independent bone.

The Sphenoid Bone

The multicomposite sphenoid bone has up to 19 intramembranous and endochondral ossification centers. Its central body, the basisphenoid, derives from the basicranial cartilage whereas its wings and pterygoid plates have both cartilaginous and intramembranous ossification centers.

The sphenoid body is derived from presphenoid and postsphenoid (basisphenoid) centers. A single median and two paired presphenoid ossification centers arise in the 4th month post conception in the mesethmoid portion of the tuberculum sellae. The postsphenoid bone, arising from two sets of paired centers in the basisphenoid cartilage on either side of the upwardly projecting hypophysial (Rathke's) pouch during the 4th month, forms the sella turcica, the dorsum sellae, and the basisphenoid (in which the notochord terminates). Coalescence of the ossification centers obliterates the orohypophysial track; the persistence of the track as a craniopharyngeal canal in the sphenoid body gives rise to craniopharyngeal tumors.

Endochondral ossification centers for the greater wings of the sphenoid appear in the alisphenoid cartilages and in the orbitosphenoid cartilages for the lesser wings. Also, intramembranous ossification centers appear in the 8th week post conception for parts of the greater wings and for the medial and lateral pterygoid plates.

The medial pterygoid plates ossify endochondrally from secondary cartilages in their hamular processes. In many fetuses, the pterygoid hamulus is a distinct, fully ossified bone at birth; it is, with the alisphenoid, the first sphenoidal elements to ossify (early in the 8th week). The hamulus is initially demarcated by a suture from the medial pterygoid plate.

Adjacent to the projecting cranial end of the basisphenoid are the paired (initially separate) sphenoidal conchae (Bertin's bones), which are incorporated into the sphenoid body postnatally and into which the sphenoidal sinuses later invaginate.

The midsphenoidal synchondrosis between the pre- and postsphenoid fuses shortly before birth. In most mammals other than man, this synchondrosis fuses late postnatally or not at all. The basisphenoid and alisphenoids are still separated at birth by mixed combined cartilaginous/ligamentous articulations. The basisphenoid articulates chondrally with the basioccipital and ligamentously with the petrosal bone. Normally, the spheno-occipital synchondrosis fuses in adolescence (see p. 99); its premature fusion in infancy results in a depressed nasal bridge and the "dished" face that characterizes many craniofacial anomalies.

THE CRANIAL BASE AND CRANIAL-BASE ANGULATION

The chondrocranium is important as a shared junction between the neurocranial and facial skeletons; its endocranial surface relates to the brain whereas its ectocranial aspect responds to the pharynx and facial complex and their muscles. Compared with the calvaria and face, the cranial base is relatively stable during growth, providing some basis against which the growth of the latter skull elements can be compared. The extremely rapid growth of the neurocranium, particularly the calvaria, contrasts with the slower and more prolonged growth of the facial skeleton. The chondrocranial base of the newborn skull is smaller than the calvarial desmocranial part, which extends beyond the base laterally and posteriorly. The relative stability of the chondrocranium maintains the early established relationships of the blood vessels, cranial nerves, and spinal cord portion that run through it.

The central region of the cranial base is composed of prechordal parts (located rostrally) and chordal parts that meet at an angle at the hypophysial fossa (sella turcica). The lower angle, formed by lines from nasion to sella to basion in the sagittal plane (Fig. 8–7), is initially highly obtuse: approximately 150° in the 4-week-old embryo (precartilage stage). It flexes to approximately 130° in the 7- to 8-week-old embryo (cartilage stage) and becomes more acute (115° to 120°) at 10 weeks (preossification stage). Between 6 and 10 weeks, the whole head is raised by extension of the neck, lifting the face from the thorax (see Fig. 10–4 in Chapter 10). This head extension is concomitant with palatal fusion. At the time of ossification of the cranial base (between 10 to 20 weeks), the cranial-base angle widens to between 125° and 130° and maintains this angulation postnatally. As the chondrocranium retains its preossification acute flexure in anencephaly, the flattening of the cranial base is probably caused by rapid growth of the brain during the fetal period.

The growth of the cranial base is highly uneven, in keeping with the highly irregular shape it develops to accommodate the undulating ventral surface of the brain. The uneven growth of the parts of the brain is reflected in the adaption of related parts of the cranial base as compartments or cranial fossae. The diencephalon is the most precocious in growth, the telencephalon is next, and the rhombencephalon (with cerebellum) is slowest in growth. The anterior and posterior parts of the cranial base, demarcated at the sella turcica, grow at different rates. Between the 10th and 40th weeks post conception, the anterior

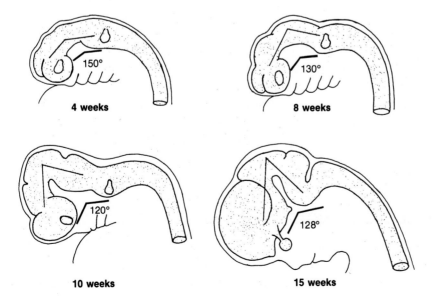

Figure 8–7 The mesencephalic flexure angles within the brain (light angulated lines) and the cranial base angles (heavy angulated lines) at various ages.

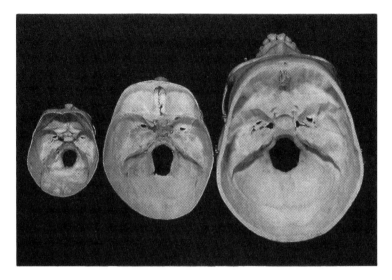

Figure 8–8 The cranial bases of a neonate (left), a 1-year-old child (center), and an adult (right), demonstrating the relatively small amount of growth in the brain stem area (sella turcica, clivus, and foramen magnum) compared with the enormous expansion of the surrounding parts. Note also the thickening of the calvarial bones from infancy to adulthood and the beginning of development of the diploë in the 1-year-old skull.

cranial base increases its length and width sevenfold, but the posterior cranial base grows only fivefold. Growth of the central ventral axis or the brain (the brain stem) and of the related body of the sphenoid and basioccipital bones is slow, providing a comparatively stable base. The anterior, middle, and posterior fossae of the cranial floor (related respectively to the frontal and temporal lobes of the cerebrum and to the cerebellum) expand enormously around this base, in keeping with the exuberant efflorescence of these parts of the brain (Figs. 8–8 and 8–9).

Expansion of the cranial base takes place as a result of (1) the growth of the cartilage remnants of the chondrocranium that persist between the bones and (2) the expansive forces that emanate from the growing brain (a capsular func-

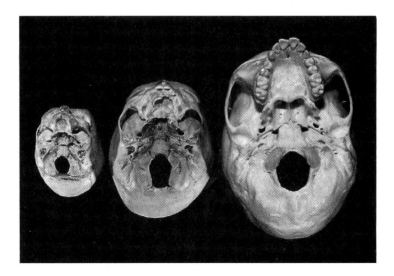

Figure 8–9 The skull bases of a neonate (left), a 1-year-old child (center), and an adult (right), demonstrating the extent of anterior facial growth from the landmark foramen magnum.

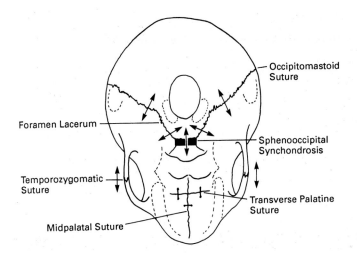

Figure 8–10 Directions of growth of cranial-base bones at suture sites, accounting for the multidirectional expansion of the cranial base.

tional matrix), displacing the bones at the suture lines (Fig. 8–10). By their interstitial growth, the interposed cartilages (synchondroses) can separate the adjacent bones as appositional bone growth adds to their sutural edges. Thus, the growth of the bones within the ventral midline (the cribriform plate of the ethmoid, the presphenoid, the basisphenoid, and the basioccipital bones) contributes to the growth of the cranial base. The cartilages between these bones contribute variably to cranial elongation and lateral expansion. Growth in the anteroposterior length of the anterior cranial fossa depends on growth at the sphenofrontal, frontoethmoidal, and sphenoethmoidal sutures. The last two sutures cease contributing to sagittal-plane growth after the age of 7 years. The internal surfaces of the frontal bone and cribriform plate cease remodeling at about 4 years of age, thereby becoming "stable" from about 6 to 7 years of age. Further growth of the anterior cranial base (anterior to the foramen caecum) is associated with expansion of the developing frontal air sinuses.

Postnatal growth in the spheno-occipital synchondrosis is the major contributor to growth of the cranial base, persisting into early adulthood. This prolonged growth period allows for continued posterior expansion of the maxilla to accommodate future erupting molar teeth and provides space for the growing nasopharynx. The spheno-occipital synchondrosis is the last of the synchondroses to fuse, beginning on its cerebral surface at 12 to13 years of age in girls and 14 to 15 years of age in boys; ossification of the external aspect is complete by 20 years of age.

Prenatally, this synchondrosis is not a major growth site. Postnatally, greater bone deposition occurs on the occipital than on the sphenoidal side of the synchondrosis, which proliferates interstitially in its midzone. Continued growth of the inferior aspect of the synchondrosis after the fusion of its superior (cerebral) surface would result in an upward and backward displacement of the basiocciput relative to the sphenoid, tending to flatten the spheno-occipital angle and thus, the cranial base. This tendency is counteracted by internal resorption of the clivus, thereby maintaining a fairly constant spheno-occipital angle during growth.

In addition to proliferative synchondrosal growth, the cranial base undergoes selective remodeling by resorption and deposition. The clivus, while resorbing on its cerebral surface, shows apposition on the nasopharyngeal (inferior) surface of the basioccipital bone and the anterior margin of the foramen magnum; thus, it can continue to lengthen after closure of the spheno-occipital synchondrosis. To maintain the size of the foramen magnum, resorption occurs at its posterior margin. The separate squamous, condylar, and basilar parts of the occipital bone fuse together only after birth. The temporal bone is composed of separate petrous, squamous, styloid, and tympanic-ring parts at birth, when the union of these parts begins. At birth, the temporal mandibular fossa is flat and lacks an articular tubercle; the occipital condyles also are flat and will become prominent only during childhood.

During growth, marked resorption in the floors of the cranial fossae deepens these endocranial compartments, a process aided by the displacement of the floors of the fossae by sutural expansion of the lateral walls of the neurocranium. Enlargement of the sella turcica is due to remodeling of its inner contour; although its anterior wall is stable by 5 to 6 years of age, its posterior wall and (to a varying extent) its floor are resorbing until 16 to 17 years of age. Owing to the variable remodeling in the sella turcica, the reference-point sella (the center of the sella turcica) cannot be regarded as stable until well after puberty. Parts of the petrous portion of the temporal bone do not resorb and are sites of some bone deposition.

Of the main elements of the skull, the cranial base (phylogenetically the oldest portion of the skull) is the most conservative in growth. The differing areas of sutural accretion, surface deposition, and resorption of bone, and the displacement, flexing, and relative re-adjustments of the bones of the cranial base form an extremely complicated pattern of overall growth. The dependence of the juxtaposed calvaria and facial skeleton on the cranial base confers considerable significance on the latter's growth behavior in determining the final shape and size of the cranium and ultimately the morphology of the entire skull, including the occlusion of the dentition. Inadequate chondrocranial growth precludes sufficient space for the full eruption of all the teeth, particularly if the maxilla is small. This leads to the impacted eruption of the last teeth to emerge (ie, the third molars).

ANOMALIES OF DEVELOPMENT

In anencephaly, the absence of the calvaria results in cranioschisis, characterized by a short, narrow, lordotic chondrocranium, with notochordal anomalies in many cases (see Fig. 2–20 in Chapter 2).

Afflictions of cartilage growth produce a reduced cranial base with increased angulation due to loss of the flattening effects of growth of the spheno-occipital synchondrosis. This results in a "dished" deformity of the middle third of the facial skeleton, accentuated by a bulging of the neurocranium. Such diverse conditions as achondroplasia, cretinism, and Down syndrome (trisomy 21 syndrome) all produce a similar characteristic facial deformity by their inhibiting effect on chondrocranial growth. Anencephalics retain the acute cranial-base flexure typical of early fetuses; this suggests that brain growth contributes to flattening of the cranial base.

Certain forms of dental malocclusion may be related to defects of the chondrocranium that minimize the space available for the maxillary dentition.

Selected Bibliography

Declau F, Jacob W, Dorrine W, et al. Early ossification within the human fetal otic capsule: morphological and microanalytical findings. J Laryngol Otol 1989;103:1113–21.

Declau F, Jacob W, Dorrine W, Marquet J. Early bone formation in the human fetal otic capsule. A methodological approach. Acta Otolaryngol Suppl 1990;470:56–60.

Dimitriadis AS, Haritani-Kouridou A, Antoniadis K, Ekonomou L. The human skull base angle during the second trimester of gestation. Neuroradiology 1995;37:68–71.

Kjaer I, Keeling JW, Fischer-Hansen B. The prenatal human cranium—normal and pathologic development. Copenhagen: Munksgaard; 1999. p. 65–133.

Kjaer I. Radiographic determination of prenatal basicranial ossification. J Craniofac Genet Dev Biol 1990;10:113–23.

Kjaer I. Neuro-osteology. Crit Rev Oral Biol Med 1998;9:224–44.

Kjaer I, Becktor KB, Nolting D, Fischer Hansen B. The association between prenatal sella turcica morphology and notochordal remnants in the dorsum sellae. J Craniofac Genet Dev Biol 1997;17:105–11.

Kjaer I, Fischer-Hansen B. The adenohypophysis and the cranial base in early human development. J Craniofac Genet Dev Biol 1995;15:157–61.

Kjaer I, Keeling JW, Graem N. Cranial base and vertebral column in human anencephalic fetuses. J Craniofac Genet Dev Biol 1994;14:235–44.

Kjaer I, Keeling JW, Graem N. Midline maxillofacial skeleton in human anencephalic fetuses. Cleft Palate Craniofac J 1994;31:250–6.

Kjaer I, Keeling JW, Reintoft I, et al. Pituitary gland and sella turcica in human trisomy 21 fetuses related to axial skeletal development. Am J Med Genet 1998;80:494–500.

Krmpotic-Nemanic J, Padovan I, Vinter I, Jalsovec D. Development of the cribriform plate and of the lamina mediana. Anat An 1998; 180:555–9.

Krmpotic Nemanic J, Vinter I, Kelovic Z. Ossicula bertini in human adults. Anat An 1998;180:55–7.

Lee SK, Kim YS, Jo YA, et al. Prenatal development of cranial base in normal Korean fetuses. Anat Rec 1996;246:524–34.

Marin-Padilla M. Cephalic axial skeletal-neural dysraphic disorders: embryology and pathology. Can J Neurol Sci 1991;18:153–69.

Molsted K, Kjaer I, Dahl E. Cranial base in newborns with complete cleft lip and palate: radiographic study. Cleft Palate Craniofac J 1995;32:199–205.

Ricciardelli FJ. Embryology and anatomy of the cranial base. Clin Plast Surg 1995; 22:361–72.

Ronning O. Basicranial synchondroses and the mandibular condyle in craniofacial growth. Acta Odontol Scand 1995;53:162–6.

Seirsen B, Jakobsen J, Skovgaard LT, Kjaer I. Growth in the external cranial base evaluated on human dry skulls, using nerve canal openings as references. Acta Odontol Scand 1997;55:356–64.

9 FACIAL SKELETON

NORMAL DEVELOPMENT

The face may be divided approximately into thirds (the upper, middle, and lower) approximately by the horizontal planes passing through the pupils of the eyes and the rima oris. The three parts correspond generally to the embryonic frontonasal, maxillary, and mandibular prominences, respectively (see p. 33). The upper third of the face is predominantly of neurocranial composition, with the frontal bone of the calvaria primarily responsible for the

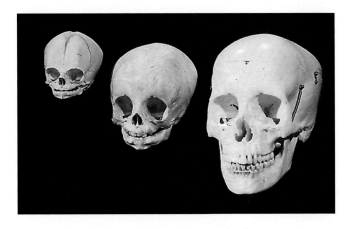

Figure 9–1 Neonatal (left), 1-year-old (center), and adult (right) skulls, illustrating the relative growth of the face and neurocranium. Note the enormous expansion of the face in the adult relative to the neonate. Note the midmandibular and frontal sutures in the neonate skull.

forehead. The middle third is the most complex skeletally, composed partly of the cranial base and incorporating both the nasal extension of the upper third and part of the masticatory apparatus (including the maxillary dentition). The lower third of the face completes the masticatory apparatus, being composed skeletally of the mandible and its dentition (see Chapter 12).

The upper third of the face initially grows the most rapidly, in keeping with its neurocranial association and the precocious development of the frontal lobes of the brain. It is also the first to achieve its ultimate growth potential, ceasing to grow significantly after 12 years of age. In contrast, the middle and lower thirds

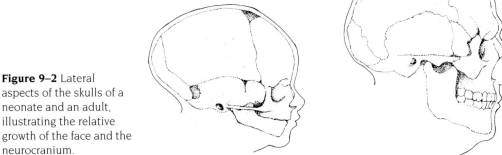

Figure 9–2 Lateral aspects of the skulls of a neonate and an adult, illustrating the relative growth of the face and the neurocranium.

TABLE 9–1 Intramembranous Ossification Centers

Bone	Site and Number of Ossification Centers		Initial Appearance
	Primary	*Secondary*	
Frontal	Superciliary arch (2)		8 weeks
		Trochlear fossa (2)	8.5 weeks
		Zygomatic process (2)	9 weeks
		Nasal spine (2)	10–12 yr
Parietal	Eminence (2)		8 weeks
Occipital (interparietal)	Supranuchal squamous (medial) (2)		8 weeks
		Supranuchal squamous (lateral) (2)	12 weeks
Temporal (desmocranial portion)	Squamous/zygomatic (1)		8 weeks
	Tympanic ring (4)		12 weeks
Nasal	Central (1)		8 weeks
Lacrimal	Central (1)		8–12 weeks
Maxilla	Body (1)		7 weeks
		Zygomatic (1)	8 weeks
		Orbitonasal (1)	8 weeks
		Nasopalatine (1)	8 weeks
Premaxilla	Intermaxillary (2)		7 weeks
Palatine	Junction of horizontal and perpendicular plates (1)		8 weeks
Vomer	Alae (2)		8 weeks
Mandible	Body (1)		6–7 weeks
		Coronoid, condylar (cartilage)	10–14 weeks
		Mental ossicles (cartilage)	7 mo pc
Zygomatic	Body (1)		8 weeks

pc = post conception.

grow more slowly over a prolonged period, not ceasing growth until late adolescence (Fig. 9–1). Completion of the masticatory apparatus by eruption of the third molars (at 18 to 25 years of age) marks the cessation of growth of the lower two-thirds of the face (Fig. 9–2).

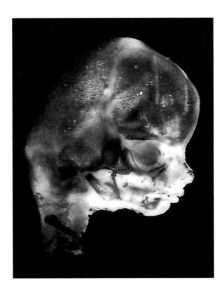

Figure 9–3 Head of a 16-week-old fetus, stained with alizarin red and alcian blue and cleared to show the extent of ossification of the bones. (Courtesy of Dr. V. H. Diewert)

EMBRYOLOGY

The facial bones develop intramembranously from ossification centers in the neural crest mesenchyme of the embryonic facial prominences (see Fig. 9–3 and Table 9–1). An epithelial-mesenchymal interaction between the ectomesenchyme of the facial prominences and the overlying ectodermal epithelium is essential for the differentiation of the facial bones.

The ossification centers for the upper third of the face are those of the frontal bone, which also contributes to the anterior part of the neurocranium. As the frontal bone is also a component of the calvaria, details of its ossification are given in Chapter 7 (see p. 83).

In the frontonasal prominence, intramembranous single ossification centers appear in the 8th week post conception for each of the nasal and lacrimal bones in the membrane covering the cartilaginous nasal capsule. The embryonic facial maxillary prominences develop numerous intramembranous ossification centers. The first centers to appear, early in the 8th week, are those for the medial pterygoid plates of the sphenoid bone and for the vomer. The ossification center for the medial pterygoid plate first appears in a nodule of secondary cartilage that forms the pterygoid hamulus; however, subsequent ossification of this plate is intramembranous. Further intramembranous centers develop for the greater wing of the sphenoid (in addition to its endochondral alisphenoidal center) and the lateral pterygoid plate. Bony fusion of the medial and lateral pterygoid plates takes place in the 5th month post conception. (For other details of sphenoid bone development, see Chapter 8, p. 96). Single ossification centers appear for each of the palatine bones, and two centers appear bilaterally for the vomer in the maxillary mesenchyme surrounding the cartilaginous nasal septum in the 8th week post conception. (For further details of vomer development, see Chapter 8, p. 91).

A primary intramembranous ossification center appears for each maxilla in the 7th week, at the termination of the infraorbital nerve just above the canine tooth dental lamina. Secondary zygomatic, orbitonasal, nasopalatine, and intermaxillary ossification centers appear and fuse rapidly with the primary centers.

The two intermaxillary ossification centers generate the alveolar ridge and primary palate region that is homologous with the premaxilla in other mammals. In humans, this area encloses the four maxillary incisor teeth; in the neonate, it is demarcated by a lateral fissure from the incisive foramen to the area between the lateral incisor and canine teeth and forms the so-called os incisivum. This bone disappears as a separate entity by fusion of the fissure in the first postnatal year.

Single ossification centers appear for each of the zygomatic bones and the squamous portions of the temporal bones in the 8th week post conception. In the lower third of the face, the mandibular prominences develop bilateral single intramembranous centers for the mandible and four minute centers for the tympanic ring of the temporal bone.

GROWTH

The attachment of the facial skeleton anteroinferiorly to the calvarial base determines the chondrocranial influence on facial growth. The sites of attachment are clearly defined by the pterygomaxillary fissure and the pterygopalatine fossa between the sphenoid bone of the calvarial base and the maxillary and palatine bones of the posterior aspect of the face. The zygomatic bone is attached to the calvarial skeleton at the temporozygomatic and the frontozygomatic sutures. The maxillary and nasal bones of the anterior aspect are attached to the calvaria at the frontomaxillary and frontonasal sutures. The interposition of three sets of space-occupying sense organs between the neural and facial skeletons complicates the attachments of these two skull components to each other and influences the growth of the facial skeleton in particular. The eye, the nasal cavity, the nasal septum, and the external ear, situated along the approximate boundaries of the upper and middle thirds of the face, act as functional matrices to some extent in determining certain aspects of the growth pattern of the face. The tongue, the teeth, and the oromasticatory musculature are similarly interposed between the middle and lower thirds of the face, and their functioning, also, influences facial skeletal growth.

The growth of the eyes provides an expanding force separating the neural and facial skeletons, particularly at the frontomaxillary and frontozygomatic sutures, thereby contributing to skull height. The eyes appear to migrate medially from their initial lateral situation in the primitive face, due to the enormous expansion of the frontal and temporal lobes of the brain in early cranial development. The forward-directed eyes of humans (and higher primates) confer a capability for stereoscopic vision and depth perception.

The eyeballs initially grow rapidly, following the neural pattern of growth and contributing to rapid widening of the fetal face. The orbits complete half their postnatal growth during the first 2 years after birth and thus appear disproportionately large in the child's face. The brain and eyeballs, growing concomitantly in a similarly rapid pattern, compete for space; the final form of the intervening orbital wall reflects mutual adjustment between these competing functional matrices. The orbital cavities attain their adult dimensions at about 7 years of age.

The nasal cavity and (in particular) the nasal septum have considerable influence in determining facial form. In the fetus, a septomaxillary ligament arising from the sides and anteroinferior border of the nasal septum and inserting into the anterior nasal spine, transmits septal growth "pull" to the maxilla. Facial growth is directed downward and forward by the septal cartilage, which expands its vertical length sevenfold between the 10th and 40th weeks post conception. At birth, the nasal cavity lies almost entirely between the orbits. Growth of the nasal septal cartilage continues (but at a decreasing rate) until the age of 6 years, lowering the nasal cavity floor below the orbits (see Fig. 9–1).

The thrust and pull created by nasal septal growth separate the frontomaxillary, frontonasal, frontozygomatic, and zygomaticomaxillary sutures to varying degrees. The growth potential of the nasal septal cartilage is clearly demonstrated in cases of bilateral cleft lip and palate: the tip of the nose, columella, philtrum, prolabium, and primary palate form a globular process that,

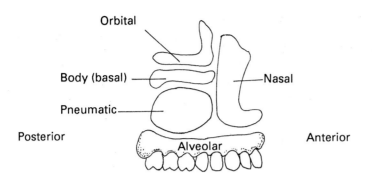

Figure 9–4 Schema of "skeletal units" of the maxilla.

freed from its lateral attachments to the maxillae, protrudes conspicuously on the face as a result of vomerine and nasal septal growth (see Fig. 3–23 in Chapter 3). This growth thrust normally dissipates into adjacent facial structures, which indicates some resistance to it. It is of interest that the nasal septum deflects from the midline during late childhood, indicating some resistance to septal growth thrust. The expansion of the eyeballs, the brain, and the spheno-occipital synchondrosal cartilage also act variously in separating the facial sutures. Furthermore, these sutures are later subjected to forces exerted by the masticatory muscles (ie, masticatory pressures transmitted through adjacent bones).

Growth of the maxilla depends on the influence of several functional matrices that act upon different areas of the bone, thus theoretically allowing its subdivision into "skeletal units" (Fig. 9–4). The "basal" body develops beneath the infraorbital nerve, later surrounding it to form the infraorbital canal. The orbital unit responds to the growth of the eyeball, the nasal unit depends upon the septal cartilage for its growth, and the teeth provide the functional matrix for the alveolar unit. The pneumatic unit reflects maxillary sinus expansion, which is more a responder than a determiner of this skeletal unit. (Development of the maxillary sinus is further described in Chapter 11, p. 123).

The complex action of these functional forces on the facial bones results in different effects on different sutures (Fig. 9–5). Thus, the temporozygomatic suture in the zygomatic arch grows predominantly in an anteroposterior horizontal direction largely due to the longitudinal growth of the brain and the

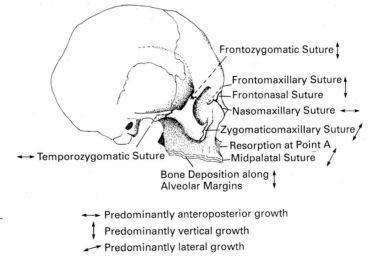

Figure 9–5 Directions of growth and resorption of the facial bones at various sites. The overall effect of the combination of these growth sites is a downward and forward displacement of the face vis-à-vis the cranial base.

spheno-occipital synchondrosal cartilage. The anteroposterior growth at the nasomaxillary sutures, creating the elevated bridge of the nose, results from anteroposterior nasal septal expansion. The frontomaxillary, frontozygomatic, frontonasal, ethmoidomaxillary, and frontoethmoidal sutures are the sites of bone growth in a largely vertical direction as a result of eyeball and nasal septal expansion. If growth of the nasal septum is defective, the height of the middle third of the face is less affected than its anteroposterior dimension, resulting in concavity of the face. Growth at the intermaxillary suture and the lateral expansion of the zygomaticomaxillary sutures by the eyes contribute to the widening of the face. In the neonate, facial width is relatively less in proportion to the neurocranium than it is in the adult. The face of the newborn is twice as broad in comparison with its height than is the adult face; it adjusts to adult proportions during the childhood years.

The overall effect of these diverse directions of growth is osseous accretion predominantly on the posterior and superior surfaces of the facial bones. Encapsulated fatty tissue, interposed between the posterosuperior surfaces of the maxilla and the cranial base (sphenoid bone), provides a compression-resisting structure. Bone deposition on the posterosuperior maxillary surface and in the region of the maxillary alveolar tuberosity displaces the maxilla away from this retromaxillary fat pad. With fat pads and the chondrocranium acting as a base against which facial bone growth takes place, the middle and (as will be seen later) lower thirds of the face move in a marked downward and slightly forward direction vis-à-vis the cranial base. Growth at these suture sites is greatest until the age of 4 years. Thereafter, these sutures function mainly as sites of fibrous union of the skull bones, allowing for adjustments brought by surface apposition and remodeling.

Remodeling takes place on all bone surfaces to adjust the bones to their new positions after displacement. Of particular interest is the deposition of bone along the alveolar margins of the maxillae (and mandible), forming incipient alveolar processes in which tooth germs develop; when tooth germs are congenitally absent, these processes fail to develop. The growth of the alveolar processes adds considerably to the vertical height of the face and to the depth of the palate and allows the concomitant expansion of the maxillary sinuses. Bone deposition on the posterior surface of the maxillary tuberosity induces corresponding anterior displacement of the entire maxilla. Eruption of teeth initially located immediately subjacent to the orbit accentuates both vertical and posterior growth of the maxillae. The growth pattern of the dental alveolar arch differs from that of the facial skeleton, being related to the sequence of tooth eruption. Resorption along the anterior surface of the bodies of the maxillae creates the supra-alveolar concavity (*point* A in orthodontic parlance), thus emphasizing the projection of the anterior nasal spine of the maxilla.

The empty space of the nasal cavity may also influence facial growth and form. Inadequate use of the nasal cavity by mouth breathing has been associated with the narrow pinched face and high-vaulted palatal arch of the adenoid facies, called thus because of a postulated association with hypertrophied pharyngeal tonsils or "adenoids." The cause-and-effect relationship (if any) of this particular (inherited?) facial form with mouth breathing has not been substantiated.

The role of the ear, as a space-occupying sense organ, in determining facial form is somewhat ambiguous and is probably minimal. The otic capsule that houses the vestibulocochlear apparatus completes its ossification from 14 centers to form the petrous temporal bone in the latter part of the 5th month and early in the 6th month of fetal life, the time at which the internal ear approaches its adult size,. The inner ear is the only organ that approaches adult size by this age. This early completion minimizes any influence on the subsequent growth of the cranial skeleton. However, the location of the inner and middle ears in the floor of the cranial cavity necessarily results in encroachment of the vestibulocochlear organ on the brain space between the middle and posterior endocranial fossae. Together with the deposition of osseous tissue on the endocranial surface of the petrous temporal bone, this infringement on brain space may cause compensatory increases of the cranial cavity in other directions.

ANOMALIES OF DEVELOPMENT

Maldevelopment of the face may arise from aberrations of morphogenesis at many levels of development and may be genetically or environmentally determined. Many congenital abnormalities originate in the maldevelopment of neural crest tissue (neurocristopathy) that gives rise to much of the skeletal and connective-tissue primordia of the face. Neural crest cells may be deficient in number, may not complete migration to their destination, or may fail in their inductive capacity or cytodifferentiation. Also, failure of ectoderm or endoderm matrix to respond to neural crest induction may give rise to facial defects.

Absence or insufficiency of neural crest ectomesenchyme in the frontonasal prominence may result in cleft lip. Deficiencies of maxillary-prominence and pharyngeal-arch ectomesenchyme (possibly because of the long path of neural crest migration) may result in absent facial bones. The clinical syndrome of mandibulofacial dysostosis (Treacher Collins syndrome), with its sunken cheeks, is due to severe hypoplasia or absence of the zygomatic bones.

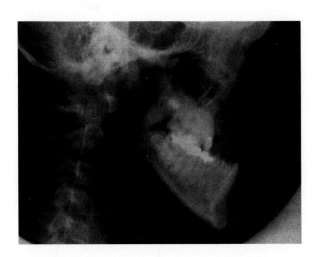

Figure 9–6 Radiograph of deficient maxillary development in a 16-year-old boy who also manifested a right-sided cleft of the lip and palate. The mandible is overgrown, exaggerating the discrepancy between the lower and middle thirds of the face.

Deficient facial bone development in anhidrotic ectodermal dysplasia, with its "dished" face, may reflect defective mechanisms of ectodermal induction by neural crest tissue. Down syndrome (trisomy 21 syndrome) features less-proclined and shortened or even absent nasal bones, accounting for the characteristic "saddle nose," and a maxilla of subnormal size. Deficient maxillary development may also be associated with clefts of the upper lip and palate (Fig. 9–6).

Incomplete brain development (holoprosencephaly) greatly influences facial formation. An extreme defect arising from holoprosencephaly is a median eye (cyclopia) (see Fig. 3–20 in Chapter 3). In normal development, the distance separating the eyes greatly influences the character of the face. A narrow interocular distance (hypotelorism) confers a sharp "foxy" appearance to the face; ocular hypertelorism, characterized by an abnormally wide interorbital distance, confers a wide-eyed appearance. This latter mild developmental defect is due to an embryological morphokinetic arrest that leaves the orbits in a fetal position, the nasal bones and cribriform plate of the ethmoid remain especially widened, and the sphenoid bone is enlarged. A more severe form of hypertelorism results in a bifid nose.

The ectomesenchymal and mesodermal deficiencies that produce these abnormalities are occasionally due to chromosomal anomalies and mutant genes, but environmental factors are involved in most cases. Facial clefts, including those afflicting the lips and palate, are components of over 250 named syndromes, many of which are of single-gene inheritance.

Unilateral defective facial development (hemifacial microsomia) produces an asymmetric face. The underdeveloped structures on the affected side are the ear, including the ear ossicles (microtia), zygomatic bone, and mandible. In addition, the parotid gland, the tongue, and the facial muscles are unilaterally defective. This condition results from a destructive hematoma emanating from the primitive stapedial artery at about the 32nd day of development.

Congenital excrescences of abnormal facial growth may occur as midline frontal or nasal masses; they include encephaloceles, gliomas, and dermoid cysts. Congenital invaginations of the face constitute dermal sinuses and fistulae. There is intracranial communication in many of these facial anomalies through defects of the cranial bones. Herniation of the intracranial contents through the frontonasal, frontoethmoidal, or frontosphenoidal complexes occurs if the foramen caecum of the frontoethmoid suture fails to close (see Fig. 7–3 in Chapter 7).

(Other defects of facial development are covered on p. 45.)

Selected Bibliography

Arnold WH, Sperber GH, Machin GA. Cranio-facial skeletal development in three human synophthalmic holoprosencephalic fetuses. Anat Anz 1998;180:45–53.

Cussenot O, Zouaoui A, Hidden G. Growth of the facial bones of the fetus. Surg Radiol Anat 1990;12:230–1.

Flugel C, Schram K, Rohen JW. Postnatal development of skull base, neuro- and viscerocranium in man and monkey: morphometric evaluation of CT scans and radiograms. Acta Anat 1993;146:71–80.

Gill PP, VanHook J, FitzSimmons J, et al. Upper face morphology of second-trimester fetuses. Early Hum Dev 1994;37:99–106.

Guis F, Ville Y, Vincent Y, et al. Ultrasound evaluation of the length of the fetal nasal bones throughout gestation. Ultrasound Obstet Gynecol 1995;5:304–7.

Kjaer I. Prenatal skeletal maturation of the human maxilla. J Craniofac Genet Dev Biol 1989;9:257–64.

Kjaer I. Correlated appearance of ossification and nerve tissue in human fetal jaws. J Craniofac Genet Dev Biol 1990;10:329–36.

Kimes KR, Mooney MP, Siegel MI, Todhunter JS. Growth rate of the vomer in normal and cleft lip and palate human fetal specimens. Cleft Palate Craniofac J 1992;29:38–42.

Lee SK, Kim YS, Lim CY, Chi JG. Prenatal growth pattern of the human maxilla. Acta Anat 1992;145:1–10.

Mandarim-de-Lacerda CA, Urania-Alves M. Growth allometry of the human face: analysis of the osseous component of the mid and lower face in Brazilian fetuses. Anat Anz 1993;175:475–9.

Nemzek WR, Brodie HA, Chong BW, et al. Imaging findings of the developing temporal bone in fetal specimens. AJNR Am J Neuroradiol 1996;17:1467–77.

Niida S, Yamanoto S, Kodama H. Variations in the running pattern of trabeculae in growing human nasal bones. J Anat 1991;179:39–41.

Piza JE, Northrop CC, Eavey RD. Neonatal mesenchyme temporal bone study: typical receding pattern versus increase in Potter's sequence. Laryngoscope 1996;107:856–864.

Radlanski RJ, Renz H, Lange S. Prenatal development of the human maxilla from 19–76 mm CRL. Ann Anat 2000;182:98.

Sandikcioglu M, Molsted K, Kjaer I. The prenatal development of the human nasal and vomeral bones. J Craniofac Genet Dev Biology 1994;14:124–34.

Siegel MI, Mooney MP, Kimes KR, Todhunter J. Developmental correlates of midfacial components in a normal and cleft lip and palate human fetal sample. Cleft Palate Craniofac J 1991;28:408–12.

10 THE PALATE

NORMAL PALATAL DEVELOPMENT

In its embryological development, the human palate passes through stages representing divisions of the oronasal chamber found in primitive crossopterygian fishes, reptiles, and early mammals. The development of internal nares or choanae marks the adoption of air-breathing by establishing

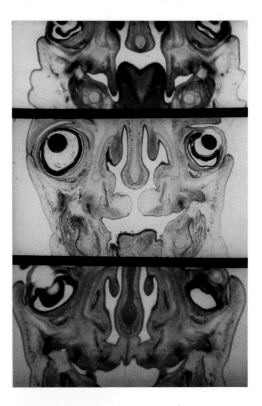

Figure 10–1 Coronally sectioned views of palate development in human embryos. Top: 54 days, vertical shelves; middle: 57 days, elevated shelves; bottom: 63 days, fused shelves with nasal septum. (Courtesy of Dr. V. Diewert and the Carnegie Embryo Collection)

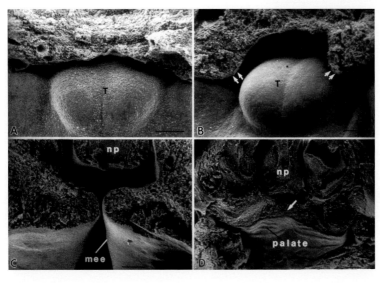

Figure 10–2 Coronal scanning electron micrographs of mouse embryos at stages of palatogenesis corresponding to human embryos. (**A**) 40 days; (**B**) 50 days; (**C**) 56 days; (**D**) 60 days. T, tongue; np, nasal prominence (septum); mee, medial-edge epithelium. (Courtesy of Dr. H. C. Slavkin)

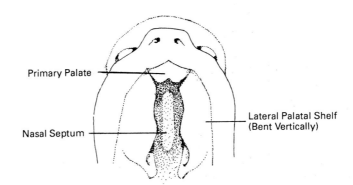

Figure 10–3
Schematic view of the three primordia of the palate in a 7½-week-old embryo.

a connection between the olfactory sacs and the stomodeum. The separation of a continuous respiratory channel (the nostrils) from an intermittently required food ingestion channel (the mouth) made possible the development of leisurely mastication without respiratory interference. This separation occurs only anteriorly, since the nasopharynx and oropharynx share a common channel posteriorly, accounting for momentary asphyxiation during swallowing. However, in the neonate and infant up to 6 months of age, concomitant breathing and swallowing occur due to the epiglottis and soft palate being in contact, maintaining a continuous airway between the nasopharynx and laryngopharynx. Milk passes on either side of this airway into the esophagus. An oropharynx develops only upon the descent of the larynx, thus separating the soft palate from the epiglottis.

The existence of an intact palate has enabled sophisticated masticatory movements and epicurian enjoyment to evolve by virtue of the taste and tex-

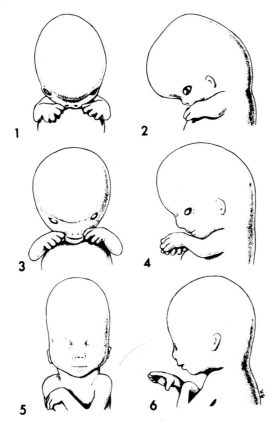

Figure 10–4 Frontal and lateral appearances of human craniofacial morphology during the late embryonic and early fetal period. 1 and 2: stage 20 embryo, crown-rump (CR) length 20 mm (× 4). 3 and 4: fetus aged 8½ weeks, CR length 35 mm (× 2). 5 and 6: fetus aged 12 weeks, CR length 80 mm (× 1). (Courtesy of Dr. V. Diewert)

ture senses embedded in the palate, accounting for the popular concept of the palate being the seat of taste. Moreover, an intact palate is quintessential for the production of normal speech. Deficiencies of palatal development will result in food and salivary spillage into the nostrils and impaired speech articulation.

The three elements that make up the secondary definitive palate—the two lateral maxillary palatal shelves and the primary palate of the frontonasal prominence—are initially widely separated due to the vertical orientation of the lateral shelves on either side of the tongue (see Figs. 3–13, 3–15, and 3–17 in Chapter 3). During the 8th week post conception, a remarkable transformation in the position of the lateral shelves takes place when they change from vertical to horizontal as a prelude to their fusion and to partitioning of the oronasal chamber (Figs. 10–1 to 10–3).

The transition from vertical to horizontal is completed within hours.* Several mechanisms have been proposed for this rapid elevation of the palatal shelves, including biochemical transformations in the physical consistency of the connective-tissue matrix of the shelves, variations in vasculature and blood flow to these structures, a sudden increase in their tissue turgor, rapid differential mitotic growth, an "intrinsic shelf-elevating force," and muscular movements. The intrinsic shelf-elevating force is chiefly generated by the accumulation and hydration of hyaluronic acid. The alignment of mesenchymal cells within the palatal shelves may serve to direct the elevating forces, while palatal mesenchymal cells are themselves contractile. The withdrawal of the embryo's face from against the heart prominence by the uprighting of the head facilitates jaw opening (Fig. 10–4). Mouth-opening reflexes have been implicated in the withdrawal of the tongue from between the vertical shelves, and pressure differences between the nasal and oral regions due to tongue muscle contraction may account for palatal-shelf elevation.

During palate closure, the mandible becomes more prognathic and the vertical dimension of the stomodeal chamber increases, but maxillary width remains stable, allowing shelf contact to occur. Also, forward growth of Meckel's cartilage relocates the tongue more anteriorly, concomitant with upper-facial elevation.

The epithelium overlying the edges of the palatal shelves is especially thickened, and their fusion upon mutual contact is crucial to intact palatal development. Fusion also occurs between the dorsal surfaces of the fusing palatal shelves and the lower edge of the midline nasal septum. The fusion seam initially forms anteriorly in the region of the hard palate, with subsequent merging in the region of the soft palate. The mechanisms of adhesive contact, fusion, and subsequent degeneration of the epithelium are not clearly understood. A combination of degenerating epithelial cells and a surface-coat accumulation of glycoproteins and desmosomes facilitates epithelial adherence between contacting palatal shelves. Only the medial-edge epithelium of the palatal shelves (in contrast to their oral and nasal surface epithelia) undergoes

---

* Shelf elevation and fusion begin a few days earlier in male than in female embryos, possibly accounting for sex differences in the incidence of cleft palate.

Figure 10–5 Lines of fusion of the embryological primordia of the palate.

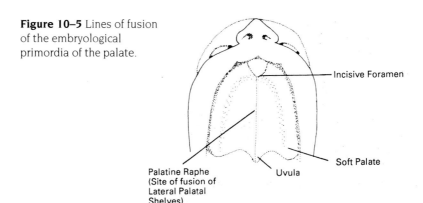

Incisive Foramen

Soft Palate

Palatine Raphe
(Site of fusion of
Lateral Palatal
Shelves)

Uvula

cytodifferentiation, involving a decline of epidermal growth factor receptors that leads to apoptotic cell death. Programmed cell death of the fusing epithelia is restricted to the periderm. Epithelial-mesenchymal transformation of medial-edge epithelial basal cells is essential to mesenchymal coalescence of the shelves. Some epithelial cells also migrate into the palatal mesenchyme, contributing to seam disruption and mesodermal confluence. The epithelium at the shelves' leading edges may contribute to failure of fusion by not breaking down after shelf approximation (leading to the formation of epithelial pearls) or by not maintaining an "adhesiveness" beyond a critical time, should palatal-shelf elevation be delayed.*

Fusion of the three palatal components initially produces a flat unarched roof to the mouth. The fusing lateral palatal shelves overlap the anterior primary palate, as indicated later by the sloping pathways of the junctional incisive neurovascular canals that carry the previously formed incisive nerves and blood vessels. The site of junction of the three palatal components is marked by the incisive papilla overlying the incisive canal. The line of fusion of the lateral palatal shelves is traced in the adult by the midpalatal suture (inclusive of the palatal portion of the intermaxillary suture and the median palatine suture between the two palatine bones) and on the surface by the midline raphe of the hard palate (Figs. 10–5 and 10–6). This fusion "seam" is minimized in the soft palate by invasion of extraterritorial mesenchyme.

Ossification of the palate proceeds during the 8th week post conception

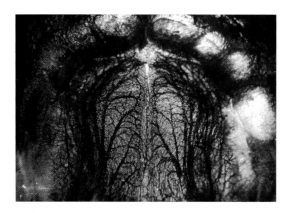

Figure 10–6 Photomicrograph of the palate of a human 6-month-old fetus. Bone has been removed by microdissection, and the arteries and capillaries have been injected with india ink. Note the midline raphe and the arterial anastomotic arcades, with only capillaries crossing over the midline. The tooth buds in the dental arch are outlined by the surrounding vascular networks. (Courtesy of Dr. William P. Maher)

---

*In birds, the medial-edge epithelium keratinizes, precluding fusion and resulting in "physiologic" cleft palate.

from the spread of bone into the mesenchyme of the fused lateral palatal shelves and from trabeculae appearing in the primary palate as "premaxillary centers," all derived from the single primary ossification centers of the maxillae. Posteriorly, the hard palate is ossified by trabeculae spreading from the single primary ossification centers of each of the palatine bones.

Midpalatal sutural structure is first evident at 10½ weeks, when an upper layer of fiber bundles develops across the midline. In infancy, the midpalatal suture in coronal section has a Y shape, and it binds the vomer with the palatal shelves. In childhood, the junction between the three bones rises into a T shape, with the interpalatal section taking a serpentine course. In adolescence, the suture becomes so interdigitated that mechanically interlocking and interstitial islets of bone are formed. Into adulthood, the palatine bone elements of the palate remain separated from the maxillary elements by the transverse palatomaxillary sutures.

Ossification does not occur in the most posterior part of the palate, giving rise to the region of the soft palate. Myogenic mesenchymal tissue of the first and fourth pharyngeal arches migrates into this faucial region, supplying the musculature of the soft palate and fauces. The tensor veli palatini is derived from the first arch, and the levator palatini, uvular, and faucial pillar muscles are derived from the fourth arch, accounting for the innervation by the first-arch trigeminal nerve of the tensor veli palatini muscle and by the fourth-arch pharyngeal plexus and vagus nerve for all the other muscles.

The tensor veli palatini is the earliest of the five palatal muscles to develop, forming myoblasts at 40 days post conception. It is followed by the palatopharyngeus (45 days), the levator veli palatini (8th week), the palatoglossus, and the uvular muscle at the 9th week; the palatoglossus, derived from the tongue musculature, attaches to the soft palate during the 11th week. The hard palate grows in length, breadth, and height, becoming an arched roof for the mouth (Fig. 10–7). The fetal palate's length increases more rapidly than its width between 7 and 18 weeks, after which the width increases

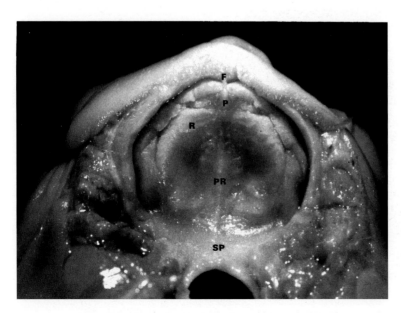

Figure 10–7 Palate and upper lip of a 22-week-old fetus. Note the midline frenulum (F), the papilla (P) overlying the incisive foramen, and the grooved alveolar arch divided into segments containing the developing tooth buds. The palatine raphe (PR) marks the site of palatal-shelf fusion. The rugae (R) become more prominent towards birth. The soft palate (SP) is extensive.

At Birth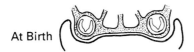

1 Year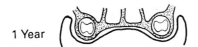

Adult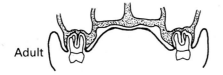

Figure 10–8 Cross-sectional views of the palate at various ages. Note the increasing depth of the palatal arch concomitant with tooth eruption.

faster than the length. In early prenatal life, the palate is relatively long, but from the 4th month post conception, it widens as a result of midpalatal sutural growth and appositional growth along the lateral alveolar margins. At birth, the length and breadth of the hard palate are almost equal. The postnatal increase in palatal length is due to appositional growth in the maxillary tuberosity region and, to some extent, at the transverse maxillopalatine suture.

Growth at the midpalatal suture ceases between 1 and 2 years of age, but no synostosis occurs to signify its cessation.* Growth in the width of the midpalatal suture is larger in its posterior than in its anterior part, so that the posterior part of the nasal cavity widens more than its anterior part. Obliteration of the midpalatal suture may start in adolescence, but complete fusion is rarely found before 30 years of age. The timing and degree of fusion of this suture varies greatly.

Lateral appositional growth continues until 7 years of age, by which time the palate achieves its ultimate anterior width. Posterior appositional growth continues after lateral growth has ceased, so that the palate becomes longer than wider during late childhood. During infancy and childhood, bone apposition also occurs on the entire inferior surface of the palate, accompanied by concomitant resorption from the superior (nasal) surface. This bone remodeling results in descent of the palate and enlargement of the nasal cavity. Nasal capacity must increase to keep pace with the increasing respiratory requirements engendered by general body growth. A fundamental drive in facial growth is the provision of an adequate nasal capacity; if the need is not met, this drive is diverted to the mouth to maintain respiration.

The appositional growth of the alveolar processes contributes to the deepening and widening of the vault of the bony palate, adding to the height and breadth of the maxillae at the same time (Fig. 10–8). The lateral alveolar processes help to form an anteroposterior palatal furrow; together with a concave floor produced by a tongue curled from side to side, this results in a

*The retention of a syndesmosis in the midpalatal suture into adulthood, even after growth has normally ceased at this site, permits the application of expansion. Forceful separation of the suture by an orthodontic appliance re-institutes compensatory bone growth at this site, expanding palatal width.

palatal tunnel ideally suited to receive a nipple. A variable number of transverse palatal rugae develop in the mucosa covering the hard palate. They appear even before palatal fusion, which occurs at 56 days post conception. The rugae, which are most prominent in the infant, hold the nipple while it is being milked by the tongue. The anterior palatal furrow is well marked during the 1st year of life (ie, the active suckling period) and normally flattens out into the palatal arch after 3 to 4 years of age when suckling has been discontinued. Persistent thumb or finger sucking may cause the accentuated palatal furrow to be retained into childhood.

ANOMALIES OF PALATAL DEVELOPMENT

Successful fusion of the three embryonic components of the palate involves complicated synchronization of shelf movements with growth and withdrawal of the tongue and with growth of the mandible and head. The mis-timing of any of these critical events, due to environmental agents or to genetic predisposition, results in the failure of fusion, leading to clefts of the palate.

The entrapment of epithelial rests or pearls in the line of fusion of the palatal shelves (particularly the midline raphe of the hard palate) may give rise later to median palatal "rest" cysts. A common superficial expression of these epithelial entrapments is the development of epithelial cysts or nodules, known as *Epstein's pearls*, along the median raphe of the hard palate and at the junction of the hard and soft palates. Small mucosal gland retention cysts (Bohn's nodules) may occur on the buccal and lingual aspects of the alveolar ridges, and dental lamina cysts composed of epithelial remnants of this lamina may develop on the crests of the alveolar ridges. All these superficial cysts of the palate in the newborn usually disappear by the 3rd postnatal month. An anterior midline maxillary cyst developing in the region of the primary palate cannot be of fissural origin but is a nasopalatine duct cyst encroaching anteriorly into the palate. Cysts are rare in the soft palate because of the mesenchymal merging of the shelves in this region although submucous clefts may occur.

Delayed elevation of the palatal shelves from the vertical to the horizontal (see p. 42 and Fig. 3–17 in Chapter 3) while the head is growing continuously results in a widening gap between the shelves so that they cannot meet and therefore cannot fuse. This leads to clefting of the palate when they eventually do become horizontal. Other causes of cleft palate are defective shelf fusion, failure of medial-edge epithelial cell death, possible postfusion rupture, and failure of mesenchymal consolidation and differentiation.

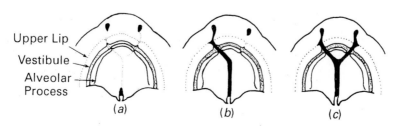

Upper Lip
Vestibule
Alveolar Process

(a)   (b)   (c)

Figure 10–9 Variations in palatal clefting: (a) bifid uvula; (b) unilateral cleft palate and lip; (c) bilateral cleft palate and lip.

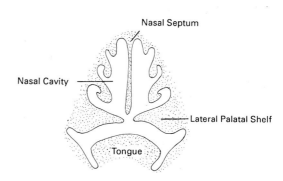

Figure 10–10 Schematic coronal section through a bilaterally cleft palate with an oral opening into both nasal cavities.

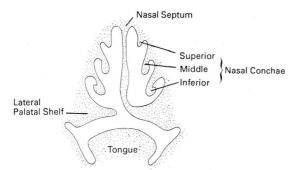

Figure 10–11 Schematic coronal section through a unilateral cleft palate with an oral opening into one nasal cavity only.

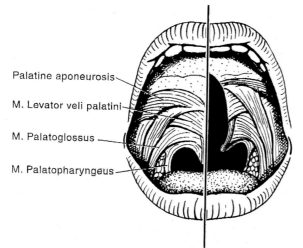

Figure 10–12 Muscle disposition in a cleft palate. Left half depicts a normal palate; right half depicts a cleft palate. M., musculus.

The least severe form of cleft palate is the relatively common bifid uvula. Increasingly severe clefts always incur posterior involvement, the cleft advancing anteriorly in contradistinction to the direction of normal fusion. The lines of fusion of the lateral palatal shelves with the primary palate dictate the diversion from the midline of a severe palatal cleft anteriorly to the right, to the left, or (in rare instances) to both. If the cleft involves the alveolar arch, it usually passes between the lateral incisor and canine teeth. Such severe clefting of the palate may or may not be associated with unilateral or bilateral cleft upper lip; the two conditions are determined independently. The vertical nasal septum may fuse with the left, the right, or (in cases of severe cleft palate) neither palatal shelf (Figs. 10–10 and 10–11).

Clefts of the soft palate alone cause varying degrees of speech difficulty and minor swallowing problems because of the inability to close off the oropharynx completely from the nasopharynx during these pharyngeal functions (Fig. 10–12). Clefts of the hard palate, which invariably include soft-palate clefts, give rise to feeding problems, particularly in infants, in whom the vacuum- producing sucking processes demand an intact hard palate. Spillage of food into the nasal fossa(e) is symptomatic of feeding difficulties. Such infants require early reparative surgery and/or obturator fitting to maintain good nutrition and to aid the development of correct enunciation. Cleft palate is a feature of a number of congenital-defect syndromes, including mandibulofacial dysostosis (Treacher Collins syndrome), micrognathia (Pierre Robin syndrome), and orodigitofacial dysostosis syndrome. The palate is narrower, shorter, and lower than normal in Down syndrome (trisomy 21) although it is often described as having a high midline elevation but being horizontally flattened laterally along the alveolar ridges, creating a "steeple palate." A highly arched palate is also characteristic of Marfan syndrome (an inherited disorder manifesting skeletal and cardiovascular anomalies), in which hyperchondroplasia is a feature, but (paradoxically) with a short nasal septal cartilage. Cleidocranial dysostosis, a congenital defect of intramembranous bones, also manifests a highly arched palate with or without a cleft. Other congenital conditions displaying a highly arched palate are craniofacial dysostosis (Crouzon syndrome), acrocephalosyndactyly (Apert syndrome), progeria, Turner syndrome (XO sex chromosome complement), and oculodentodigital dysplasia.

A fairly common genetic anomaly of the palate is a localized midpalatal overgrowth of bone of varying size, known as a *torus palatinus*. This may enlarge in adulthood, and although it does not directly influence dental occlusion, it may interfere, if prominent, with the seating of a removable orthodontic appliance or upper denture.

Selected Bibliography

Arnold WH, Rezwani T, Baric I. Location and distribution of epithelial pearls and tooth buds in human fetuses with cleft lip and palate. Cleft Palate Craniofac J 1998;35:359–65.

Barrow JR, Capecchi MR. Compensatory defects associated with mutations in Hoxa 1 restore normal palatogenesis to Hoxa 2 mutants. Development 1999;126:5011–26.

Behrents RG, Harris EF. The premaxillary-maxillary suture and orthodontic mechanotherapy. Am J Orthod Dentofacial Orthop 1991;99:1–6.

Citterio HL, Gaillard DA. Expression of transforming growth factor alpha (TGF alpha), epidermal growth factor receptor (EGF-R) and cell proliferation during human palatogenesis: an immunohistochemical study. Int J Dev Biol 1994;38:499–505.

Cohen SR, Chen L, Trotman CA, Burdi AR. Soft-palate myogenesis: a developmental field paradigm. Cleft Palate Craniofac J 1993;30:441–6.

Del Santo M Jr, Minarelli AM, Liberti EA. Morphological aspects of the mid-palatal suture in the human foetus: a light and scanning electron microscopy study. Eur J Orthod 1998;20:93–9.

Diewert VM. Craniofacial growth during human secondary palate formation and potential relevance of experimental cleft palate observations. J Craniofac Genet Dev Biol Suppl 1986;2:267–76.

Fitchett JE, Hay ED. Medial edge epithelium transforms to mesenchyme after embryonic palatal shelves fuse. Dev Biol 1989;131:455–74.

Greene RM, Linask KK, Pisano MM, et al. Transmembrane and intracellular signal tranduction during palatal ontogeny. J Craniofac Genet Dev Biol 1991;11:262–76.

Harris MJ, Juriloff DM, Peters CE. Disruption of pattern formation in palatal rugae in fetal mice heterozygous for first arch (Far). J Craniofac Genet Dev Biol 1990;10:363–71.

Kimes KR, Mooney MP, Siegel MI, Todhunter JS. Size and growth rate of the tongue in normal and cleft lip and palate human fetal specimens. Cleft Palate Craniofac J 1991;28:212–6.

Kjaer I. Human prenatal palatal closure related to skeletal maturity of the jaws. J Craniofac Genet Dev Biol 1989;9:265–70.

Kjaer I. Human prenatal palatal shelf elevation related to craniofacial skeletal maturation. Eur J Orthod 1992;14:26–30.

Kjaer I. Mandibular movements during elevation and fusion of palatal shelves evaluated from the course of Meckel's cartilage. J Craniofac Genet Dev Biol 1997;17:80–5.

Kjaer I, Bach-Petersen S, Graem N, Kjaer T. Changes in human palatine bone location and tongue position during prenatal palatal closure. J Craniofac Genet Dev Biol 1993;13:18–23.

Kjaer I, Keeling J, Russell B, et al. Palate structure in human holoprosencephaly correlates with the facial malformation and demonstrates a new palatal developmental field. Am J Med Genet 1997;73:387–92.

Lavrin IG, Hay ED. Epithelial-mesenchymal transformation, palatogenesis and cleft palate. Angle Orthod 2000;70:181–2.

Lisson JA, Kjaer I. Location of alveolar clefts relative to the incisive fissure. Cleft Palate Craniofac J 1997;34:292–6.

Malek R. Cleft Lip and Palate. London: Martin Dunitz Ltd; 2000.

Millard DR Jr. Embryonic rationale for the primary correction of classical congenital clefts of the lip and palate. Ann Coll Surg Eng 1994;76:150–60.

Nijo BJ, Kjaer I. The development and morphology of the incisive fissure and the transverse palatine suture in the human fetal palate. J Craniofac Genet Dev Biol 1993;13:24–34.

Revelo B, Fishman LS. Maturational evaluation of ossification of the midpalatal suture. Am J Orthod Dentofacial Orthop 1994;105:282–92.

Rude FP, Anderson L, Conley D, Gasser RF. Three-dimensional reconstructions of the primary palate region in normal human embryos. Anat Rec 1994; 238:108–13.

Shapira Y, Lubit E, Kuftinec MM, Borell G. The distribution of clefts of the primary and secondary palates by sex, type, and location. Angle Orthod 1999;69:523–8.

Shaw WC, Simpson JP. Oral adhesions associated with cleft lip and palate and lip fistulae. Cleft Palate J 1980;17:127–31.

Shuler CF, Halpern DE, Guo Y, Sank AC. Medial edge epithelium fate traced by cell lineage analysis during epithelial-mesenchymal transformation in vivo. Dev Biol 1992;154:318–30.

Silau AM, Njio B, Solow B, Kjaer I. Prenatal sagittal growth of the osseous components of the human palate. J Craniofac Genet Dev Biol 1994; 14:252–6.

11 PARANASAL SINUSES

NORMAL DEVELOPMENT

The four sets of paranasal sinuses—maxillary, sphenoidal, frontal, and eth-moidal—begin their development at the end of the 3rd month post conception as outpouchings of the sphenoethmoidal recesses and the mucous membranes of the middle and superior nasal meatus. The early paranasal sinuses expand into the cartilage walls and roof of the nasal fossae by growth of mucous membrane sacs (primary pneumatization) into the maxillary, sphenoid, frontal, and ethmoid bones. The sinuses enlarge into bone (secondary pneumatization) from their initial small outpocketings, always retaining communication with the nasal fossae through ostia (Fig. 11–1).

Pneumatization of the paranasal bones occurs at different times and even varies between the sides. The maxillary sinus starts first, at 10 weeks post conception, developing from the middle meatus by primary pneumatization into the ectethmoid cartilage. Secondary pneumatization into the ossifying maxilla starts in the 5th month in this most precocious of the sinuses, which is large enough at birth to be clinically important and radiographically identifiable. The maxillary sinus enlarges slightly faster than overall maxillary growth, by bone resorption of the maxilla's internal walls (except medially). Sinus expansion causes resorption of cancellous bone except on the medial wall, where internal bone resorption is matched by opposing nasal surface resorption, thereby enlarging the nasal cavity. The rapid and continuous downward growth of this sinus after birth brings its walls in close proximity to the roots of the maxillary cheek teeth and brings its floor below its osteal opening. As each

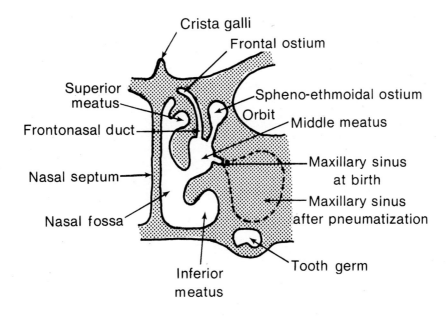

Figure 11–1 Coronal sectional schema of paranasal sinuses.

tooth erupts, the vacated bone becomes pneumatized by the expanding maxillary sinus, whose floor descends from its prenatal level above the nasal floor to its adult level below the nasal floor. In adulthood, the roots of the molar teeth commonly project into the sinus lumen. The maxillary sinus averages 7 mm in length and 4 mm in height and width at birth and expands approximately 2 mm vertically and 3 mm anteroposteriorly each year.

The sphenoidal sinuses start developing at 4 months post conception by constricting the posterosuperior portion of the sphenoethmoid recess and thus bypassing primary pneumatization. The recess is between the sphenoidal conchae (Bertin's bones) and the sphenoid body. Secondary pneumatization occurs at 6 to 7 years, into the sphenoid and into the basisphenoid bones later. The sinus continues growing in early adulthood and may invade the wings and (rarely) the pterygoid plates of the sphenoid bone.

Ethmoid air cells from the middle and superior meatus and sphenoethmoid recess invade the ectethmoid nasal capsule (primary pneumatization), from the 4th month post conception. Secondary pneumatization occurs between birth and 2 years as groups of 3 to 15 air cells grow irregularly to form the ethmoid labyrinth (Fig. 11–2). The most anterior ethmoidal cells grow upward into the frontal bone; they may form the frontal sinuses, retaining their origin from the middle meatus of the nose as the frontonasal duct. The ethmoidal air cells may also expand into the sphenoid, lacrimal, or even maxillary bones (extramural sphenoidal, lacrimal, and maxillary sinuses).

The frontal sinuses start as mucosal invaginations (primary pneumatization) in the frontal recess of the middle meatus of the nasal fossa at 3 to 4 months post conception, but they do not invade the frontal bone (secondary pneumatization) until between 6 months and 2 years postnatally and are not visible radiographically before 6 years of age. They grow upward at an extremely variable rate until puberty. All the paranasal sinuses appear to continue increasing their size into old age.

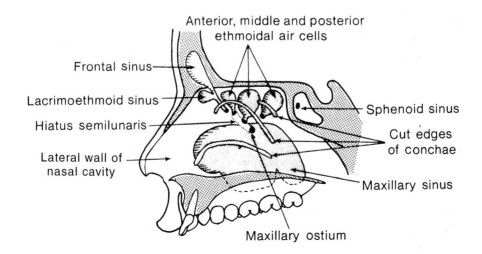

Figure 11–2 Schematic view of paranasal sinuses in the adult and their communications (ostia) with the nasal fossa.

ANOMALIES OF DEVELOPMENT

Nondevelopment of the frontal and sphenoidal sinuses is characteristic of Down (trisomy 21) syndrome. Diminution or absence of sinuses is also found in Apert syndrome (acrocephalosyndactyly). If an interfrontal (metopic) suture persists, the frontal sinuses are small or even absent.

Selected Bibliography

Arredondo de Arreola G, Lopez Serna N, de Hoyos Parra R, Arreola Salinas MA. Morphogenesis of the lateral nasal wall from 6 to 36 weeks. Otolaryngol Head Neck Surg 1996;114:54–60.

Bingham B, Wang RG, Hawke M, Kwok P. The embryonic development of the lateral nasal wall from 8 to 24 weeks. Laryngoscope 1991;101:992–7.

Gulisano M, Montella A, Orlandini SZ, Pacini P. Morphological study of fetal nasopharyngeal epithelium in man. Acta Anat 1992;144:152–9.

Helfferich F, Viragh S. Histological investigations of the nasal mucosa in human fetuses. Eur Arch Otorhinolaryngol Suppl 1997;1:S39–42.

Koppe T, Yamamoto T, Tanaka O, Nagai H. Investigations on the growth pattern of the maxillary sinus in Japanese human fetuses. Okajimas Folia Anat Jpn 1994;71:311–8.

Kubal WS. Sinonasal anatomy. Neuroimaging Clin N Am 1998;8:143–56.

Monteiro VJ, Dias MP. Morphogenic mechanisms in the development of ethmoidal sinuses. Anat Rec 1997;249:96–102.

Rossouw PE, Lombard CJ, Harris AM. The frontal sinus and mandibular growth prediction. Am J Orthod Dentofac Orthop 1991;100:542–6.

Sato I, Sunohara M, Mikami A, et al. Immunocytochemical study of the maxilla and maxillary sinus during human fetal development. Okajimas Folia Anat Jpn 1998;75:205–16.

Skladzien J, Litwin JA, Nowogrodzky-Zagorska N, Miodonski AJ. Corrosion casting study on the vasculature of nasal mucosa in the human fetus. Anat Rec 1995;242:411–6.

Smith TD, Siegel MI, Mooney MP, et al. Formation and enlargement of the paranasal sinuses in normal and cleft lip and palate human fetuses. Cleft Palate Craniofac J 1997;34:483–9.

Wake M, Takeno S, Hawke M. The early development of sino-nasal mucosa. Laryngoscope 1994;104:850–5.

Wang RG, Jiang SC. The embryonic development of the human ethmoid labyrinth from 8-40 weeks. Acta Otolaryngol 1997;117:118–22.

Wang RG, Jiang SC, Gu R. The cartilaginous nasal capsule and embryonic development of human paranasal sinuses. J Otolaryngol 1994;23:239–43.

12 THE MANDIBLE

The human mandible has no one design for life. Rather, it adapts and remodels through the seven stages of life, from the slim arbiter of things to come in the infant, through a powerful dentate machine and even weapon in the full flesh of maturity, to the pencil-thin, porcelain-like problem that we struggle to repair in the adversity of old age.

D. E. Poswillo, 1988

PRENATAL DEVELOPMENT

The cartilages and bones of the mandibular skeleton form from embryonic neural crest cells (see p. 24) that originate in the mid- and hindbrain regions of the neural folds. These cells migrate ventrally to form the mandibular (and maxillary) facial prominences, where they differentiate into bones and connective tissues.

The first structure to develop in the region of the lower jaw is the mandibular division of the trigeminal nerve that precedes the ectomesenchymal condensation forming the first (mandibular) pharyngeal arch. The prior presence of the nerve has been postulated as requisite for inducing osteogenesis by the production of neurotrophic factors. The mandible is derived from ossification of an osteogenic membrane formed from ectomesenchymal condensation at 36 to 38 days of development. This mandibular ectomesenchyme must interact initially with the epithelium of the mandibular arch before primary ossification can occur; the resulting intramembranous bone lies lateral to Meckel's cartilage of the first (mandibular) pharyngeal arch (see p. 54) (Fig. 12–1). A single ossification center for each half of the mandible arises in the 6th week post conception (the mandible and the clavicle are the first bones to begin to ossify) in the region of the bifurcation of the inferior alveolar nerve and artery into mental and incisive branches. The ossifying membrane is lateral to Meckel's cartilage and its accompanying neurovascular bundle. From the primary center below and around the inferior alveolar nerve and its incisive branch, ossification spreads upwards to form a trough for the developing teeth. The spread of the intramembranous ossification dorsally and ventrally forms the body and ramus of the mandible. Meckel's cartilage becomes surrounded and invaded by bone. Ossification stops dorsally at the site that will become the mandibular lingula, where Meckel's cartilage continues into the middle ear. The prior presence of the neurovascular bundle ensures the formation of the mandibular foramen and canal and the mental foramen.

The first pharyngeal-arch core of Meckel's cartilage almost meets its fellow of the opposite side ventrally. It diverges dorsally to end in the tympanic cavity of each middle ear, which is derived from the first pharyngeal pouch, and is surrounded by the forming petrous portion of the temporal bone. The dorsal end of Meckel's cartilage ossifies to form the basis of two of the auditory ossicles (ie, the malleus and the incus). The third ossicle (the stapes) is derived primarily from the cartilage of the second pharyngeal arch (Reichert's cartilage) (see p. 54).

Meckel's cartilage lacks the enzyme phosphatase found in ossifying cartilages, thus precluding its ossification; almost all of Meckel's cartilage disappears by the 24th week after conception. Parts transform into the sphenomandibular and anterior malleolar ligaments. A small part of its ventral end (from the mental foramen ventrally to the symphysis) forms accessory endochondral ossicles that are incorporated into the chin region of the mandible. Meckel's cartilage dorsal to the mental foramen undergoes resorption on its lateral surface at the same time as intramembranous bony trabeculae are forming immediately lateral to the resorbing cartilage. Thus, the cartilage from the mental foramen to the lingula is not incorporated into ossification of the mandible.

The initial woven bone formed along Meckel's cartilage is soon replaced by lamellar bone, and typical haversian systems are already present at the 5th month post conception. This remodeling occurs earlier than it occurs in other bones, and is thought to be a response to early intense sucking and swallowing, which stress the mandible.

Secondary accessory cartilages appear between the 10th and 14th weeks post conception to form the head of the condyle, part of the coronoid process, and the mental protuberance (see Fig. 12–1). The appearance of these secondary mandibular cartilages is dissociated from the primary pharyngeal (Meckel's) and chondrocranial cartilages. The secondary cartilage of the coronoid process develops within the temporalis muscle, as its predecessor. The coronoid accessory cartilage becomes incorporated into the expanding intramembranous bone of the ramus and disappears before birth. In the mental region, on either side of the symphysis, one or two small cartilages appear and ossify in the 7th month post conception to form a variable number of mental ossicles in the fibrous tissue of the symphysis. The ossicles become incor-

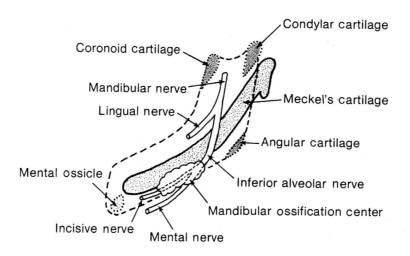

Figure 12–1 Schema of the origins of the mandible. The center of ossification is lateral to Meckel's cartilage at the bifurcation of the inferior alveolar nerve.

porated into the intramembranous bone when the symphysis menti is converted from a syndesmosis into a synostosis during the 1st postnatal year.

The condylar secondary cartilage appears during the 10th week post conception as a cone-shaped structure in the ramal region. This condylar cartilage is the primordium of the future condyle. Cartilage cells differentiate from its center, and the cartilage condylar head increases by interstitial and appositional growth. By the 14th week, the first evidence of endochondral bone appears in the condyle region. The condylar cartilage serves as an important center of growth for the ramus and body of the mandible. The nature of this growth—as primary (an initial source of morphogenesis) or secondary (compensating for functional stimulation)—is controversial, but experimental evidence indicates the need for mechanical stimuli for normal growth. By the middle of fetal life, much of the cone-shaped cartilage is replaced with bone, but its upper end persists into adulthood, acting as both growth and articular cartilage. Changes in mandibular position and form are related to the direction and amount of condylar growth. The condylar growth rate increases at puberty, peaks between 12½ and 14 years of age, and normally ceases at about 20 years of age. However, the continuing presence of the cartilage provides a potential for continued growth, which is realized in conditions of abnormal growth such as acromegaly.

POSTNATAL DEVELOPMENT

The shape and size of the diminutive fetal mandible undergo considerable transformation during its growth and development. The ascending ramus of the neonatal mandible is low and wide, the coronoid process is relatively large and projects well above the condyle, the body is merely an open shell containing the buds and partial crowns of the deciduous teeth, and the mandibular canal runs low in the body. The initial separation of the right and left bodies of the

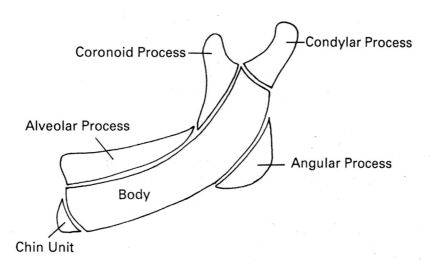

Figure 12–2 Schema of "skeletal units" of the mandible.

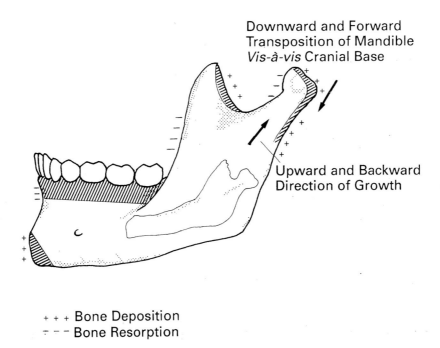

Downward and Forward
Transposition of Mandible
Vis-à-vis Cranial Base

Upward and Backward
Direction of Growth

+ + + Bone Deposition
– – – Bone Resorption

Figure 12–3 Schematic representation of mandibular growth, showing the fetal mandible superimposed upon the adult mandible.

mandible at the midline symphysis menti is gradually eliminated between the 4th and 12th months after birth, when ossification converts the syndesmosis into a synostosis, uniting the two halves.

Although the mandible appears as a single bone in the adult, it is developmentally and functionally divisible into several skeletal subunits (Fig. 12–2). The basal bone of the body forms one unit, to which are attached the alveolar, coronoid, angular, and condylar processes and the chin. The growth pattern of each of these skeletal subunits is influenced by a functional matrix that acts upon the bone: the teeth act as a functional matrix for the alveolar unit; the action of the temporalis muscle influences the coronoid process; the masseter and medial pterygoid muscles act upon the angle and ramus of the mandible; and the lateral pterygoid has some influence on the condylar process. The functioning of the related tongue and perioral muscles and the expansion of the oral and pharyngeal cavities provide stimuli for mandibular growth to reach its full potential. Of all the facial bones, the mandible undergoes the most growth postnatally and evidences the greatest variation in morphology.

Limited growth takes place at the symphysis menti until fusion occurs. The main sites of postnatal mandibular growth are at the condylar cartilages, the posterior borders of the rami, and the alveolar ridges. These areas of bone deposition largely account for increases in the height, length, and width of the mandible. However, superimposed upon this basic incremental growth are numerous regional remodeling changes that are subjected to the local functional influences involving selective resorption and displacement of individual mandibular elements (Fig. 12–3).

Direction of Condylar Growth

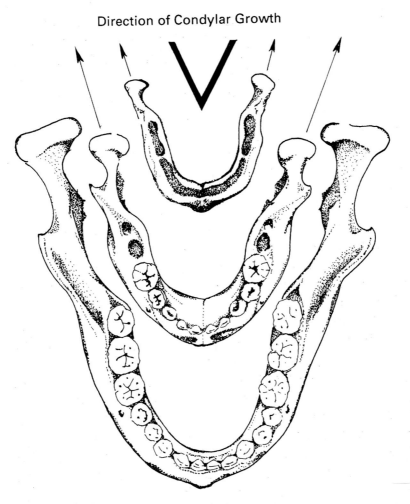

Figure 12–4 Mandibles of a neonate (top), a 4-year-old child (middle), and an adult (below), illustrating the constant width of the anterior body of the mandible as opposed to the lateral expansion of the rami with growth, indicated by arrows and the "V."

The condylar cartilage of the mandible uniquely serves as both (1) an articular cartilage in the temporomandibular joint, characterized by a fibrocartilage surface layer, and (2) a growth cartilage analogous to the epiphysial plate in a long bone, characterized by a deeper hypertrophying cartilage layer. The subarticular appositional proliferation of cartilage within the condylar head provides the basis for the growth of a medullary core of endochondral bone, on the outer surface of which a cortex of intramembranous bone is laid. The growth cartilage may act as a "functional matrix" to stretch the periosteum, inducing the lengthened periosteum to form intramembranous bone beneath it. The diverse histologic origins of the medulla and cortex are effaced by their fusion. The formation of bone within the condylar heads causes the mandibular rami to grow upward and backward, displacing the entire mandible in an opposite downward and forward direction. Bone resorption subjacent to the condylar head accounts for the narrowed condylar neck. The attachment of the lateral pterygoid muscle to this neck and the growth and action of the tongue and

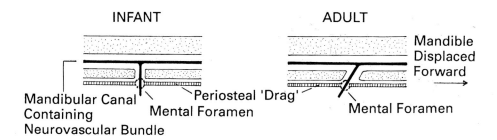

Figure 12–5 Schematic expansion of the alteration of direction of the mental foramen, from lateral in the infant to posterior in the adult, as a result of forward displacement of the mandible and "dragging" of the mental neurovascular bundle.

masticatory muscles are functional forces implicated in this phase of mandibular growth.

Any damage to the condylar cartilages restricts the growth potential and normal downward and forward displacement of the mandible, unilaterally or bilaterally, according to the side(s) damaged. Lateral deviations of the mandible and varying degrees of micrognathia and accompanying malocclusion result.

In the infant, the condyles of the mandible are inclined almost horizontally, so that condylar growth leads to an increase in the length of the mandible rather than to an increase in height. Due to the posterior divergence of the two halves of the body of the mandible (in a V shape), growth in the condylar heads of the increasingly more widely displaced rami results in overall widening of the mandibular body, which keeps pace (by remodeling) with the widening cranial base (Fig 12–4). No interstitial widening of the mandible can take place at the fused symphysis menti after the 1st year, apart from some widening by surface apposition.

Bone deposition occurs on the posterior border of the ramus, whereas concomitant resorption on the anterior border maintains the proportions of the ramus and, in effect, moves it backward in relation to the body of the mandible. This deposition and concomitant resorption extends up to the coronoid process, involving the mandibular notch, and progressively repositions the mandibular foramen posteriorly, accounting for the anterior overlying plate of the lingula. The attachment of the elevating muscles of mastication to the buccal and lingual aspects of the ramus and to the mandibular angle and coronoid process influences the ultimate size and proportions of these mandibular elements.

The posterior displacement of the ramus converts former ramal bone into the posterior part of the body of the mandible. In this manner, the body of the mandible lengthens, the posterior molar region relocating anteriorly into the premolar and canine regions. This is one means by which additional space is provided for eruption of the molar teeth, all three of which originate in the junction of the ramus and the body of the mandible. Their forward migration and posterior ramal displacement lengthen the molar region of the mandible.

The forward shift of the growing mandibular body changes the direction of the mental foramen during infancy and childhood. The mental neurovascular bundle emanates from the mandible at right angles or even a slightly forward direction at birth. In adulthood, the mental foramen (and its neurovascular content) is characteristically directed backward. This change may be ascribed to forward growth in the body of the mandible while the neurovascular bundle "drags along" (Fig. 12–5). A contributory factor may be the differing growth rates of bone and periosteum. The latter, by its firm attachment to the condyle and comparatively loose attachment to the mandibular body, grows more slowly than the body, which slides forward beneath the periosteum. The changing direction of the foramen has clinical implications in the administration of local anesthetic to the mental nerve: in infants and children, the syringe needle may be applied at right angles to the body of the mandible to enter the mental foramen whereas the needle must be applied obliquely from behind to achieve entry in the adult.

The location of the mental foramen also alters its vertical relationship within the body of the mandible from infancy to old age. When teeth are present, the mental foramen is located midway between the upper and lower borders of the mandible. In the edentulous mandible, lacking an alveolar ridge, the mental foramen appears near the upper margin of the thinned mandible (Fig. 12–6).

The alveolar process develops as a protective trough in response to the tooth buds and becomes superimposed upon the basal bone of the mandibular body. It adds to the height and thickness of the body of the mandible and is particularly manifest as a ledge extending lingually to the ramus to accommodate the third molars. The alveolar bone fails to develop if teeth are absent and resorbs in response to tooth extraction. The orthodontic movement of teeth takes place in the labile alveolar bone of both maxilla and mandible and fails to involve the underlying basal bone.

The chin, formed in part of the mental ossicles from accessory cartilages and the ventral end of Meckel's cartilage, is very poorly developed in the infant. It develops almost as an independent subunit of the mandible, influenced by sexual as well as specific genetic factors. Sex differences in the symphyseal region of the mandible are not significant until other secondary sex characteristics develop. Thus, the chin becomes significant only at adolescence, from the development of the mental protuberance and tubercles. Whereas small chins are found in adults of both sexes, very large chins are characteristically masculine. The skeletal "unit" of the chin may be an expression of the functional forces exerted by the lateral pterygoid muscles that, in pulling the mandible forward, indirectly stress the mental symphyseal region by their concomitant inward pull. Bone buttressing to resist muscle stressing, which is more powerful in the male, is expressed in the more prominent male chin. The protrusive chin is a uniquely human trait, lacking in all other primates and in hominid ancestors.

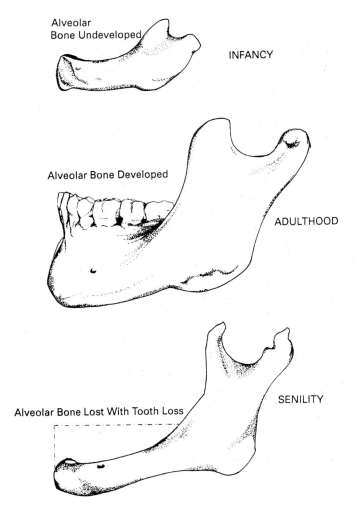

Alveolar
Bone Undeveloped

INFANCY

Alveolar Bone Developed

ADULTHOOD

SENILITY

Alveolar Bone Lost With Tooth Loss

Figure 12–6 Lateral view of the mandible in infancy, adulthood, and senility, illustrating the influence of alveolar bone on the contour of the mandibular body. Note the changing obliquity of the angle of the mandible. Note the location of the mental foramen that varies in relation to the upper border of the body of the mandible.

The mental protuberance forms by osseous deposition during childhood. Its prominence is accentuated by bone resorption in the alveolar region above it, creating the supramental concavity known as "point B" in orthodontic terminology. Underdevelopment of the chin is known as microgenia.

The torus mandibularis, a genetically determined exostosis on the lingual aspect of the body of the mandible, develops (usually bilaterally) in the canine-premolar region. This torus is unrelated to any muscle attachments or known functional matrices.

During fetal life, the relative sizes of the maxilla and mandible vary widely. Initially, the mandible is considerably larger than the maxilla, a predominance lessened later by the relatively greater development of the maxilla; by about 8 weeks post conception, the maxilla overlaps the mandible. The subsequent relatively greater growth of the mandible results in the approximately equal size of the upper and lower jaws by the 11th week. Mandibular growth lags behind maxillary growth between the 13th and 20th weeks due to a changeover from Meckel's cartilage to condylar secondary cartilage as the main growth determinant of the lower jaw. At birth, the mandible tends to be retrognathic to the maxilla although the two may be of equal size. This retrognathic condition is normally corrected early in postnatal life by rapid mandibular growth and forward displacement to establish an Angle Class I maxillomandibular relationship. Inadequate mandibular growth results in an Angle Class II relation (retrognathism), and overgrowth of the mandible produces a Class III relation (prognathism). The mandible can grow for much longer than the maxilla.

ANOMALIES OF DEVELOPMENT

In the condition of agnathia, the mandible may be grossly deficient or absent, reflecting a deficiency of neural crest tissue in the lower part of the face. Aplasia of the mandible and hyoid bone (first- and second-arch syndrome) is a rare lethal condition with multiple defects of the orbit and maxilla. Well-developed (albeit low-set) ears and auditory ossicles in this syndrome suggest ischemic necrosis of the mandible and hyoid bone occurring after the formation of the ear.

The diminutive mandible of micrognathia (Fig. 12–7) is characteristic of several syndromes, including Pierre Robin and cat's cry (cri du chat) syndromes, mandibulofacial dysostosis (Treacher Collins syndrome), progeria, Down syndrome (trisomy 21 syndrome), oculomandibulodyscephaly (Hallermann-Streiff syndrome), and Turner syndrome (XO sex chromosome complement).

A central dysmorphogenic mechanism of defective neural crest production, migration, or destruction may be responsible for the hypoplastic mandible common to these conditions. Absent or deficient neural crest tissue around the optic cup causes a "vacuum," so that the developing otic pit (normally adjacent to the second pharyngeal arch) moves cranially into first-arch territory and the ear becomes located over the angle of the mandible. Derivatives of the deficient ectomesenchyme (specifically the zygomatic, maxillary, and mandibular bones) are hypoplastic, accounting for the typical facies common to these syndromes.

In Pierre Robin syndrome, the underdeveloped mandible usually demonstrates catch-up growth in the child. In mandibulofacial dysostosis, deficiency of the mandible is maintained throughout growth. In unilateral agenesis of the mandibular ramus, the malformation increases with age. Hemifacial microsomia (Goldenhar syndrome) also becomes more severe with retarded growth.

Variations in condylar form may occur, among them the rare bifid or double condyle that results from the persistence of septa dividing the fetal condylar cartilage.

Macrognathia, producing prognathism, is usually an inherited condition, but abnormal-growth phenomena such as hyperpituitarism may produce mandibular overgrowth of increasing severity with age. Congenital hemifacial hypertrophy, evident at birth, tends to intensify at puberty. Unilateral

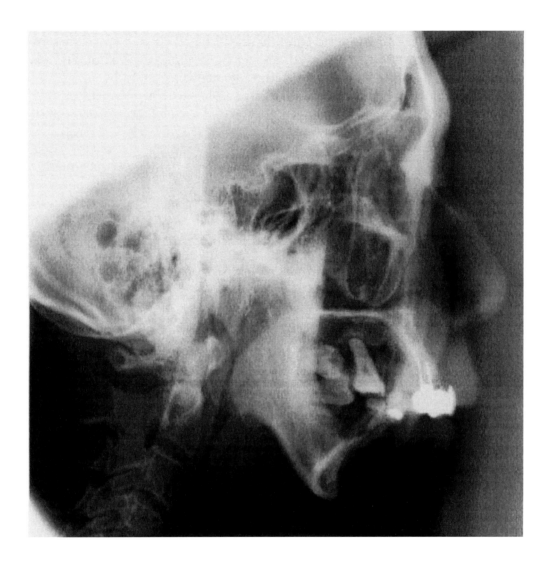

Figure 12–7 Radiograph of deficient mandibular development in a 45-year-old male. The severe micrognathia is due to mandibular condyle degeneration consequent to bilateral condylar fractures at 4 years of age, with reduction by wires still present in condyles. The temporomandibular joints are ankylosed, with dental malocclusion present. (Compare with Fig. 9–6 in Chapter 9.) (Courtesy of Dr. G. W. Raborn)

enlargement of the mandible, the mandibular fossa, and the teeth is of obscure etiology; more common is isolated unilateral condylar hyperplasia.

Selected Bibliography

Azeredo RA, Watanabe I, Liberti EA, Semprini M. The arrangement of the trabecular bone in the vestibular surface of the human fetus mandible. I. A scanning electron microscopy study (1). Bull Assoc Anat 1996;80:7–12.

Bareggi R, Narducci P, Grill V, et al. On the presence of a secondary cartilage in the mental symphyseal region of human embryos and fetuses. Surg Radiol Anat 1994;16:379–84.

Bareggi R, Sandrucci MA, Baldini G, et al. Mandibular growth rates in human fetal development. Arch Oral Biol 1995;40:119–25.

Barni T, Maggi M, Fantoni G, et al. Identification and localization of endothelin-1 and its receptors in human fetal jaws. Dev Biol 1995;169:373–7.

Ben Ami Y, von der Mark K, Franzen A, et al. Immunohistochemical studies of the extracellular matrix in the condylar cartilage of the human fetal mandible: collagens and noncollagenous proteins. Am J Anat 1991;190:157–66.

Ben-Ami Y, Lewinson D, Silbermann M. Structural characterization of the mandibular condyle in human fetuses: light and electron microscopy studies. Acta Anat 1992;145:79–87.

Ben-Ami Y, von der Mark K, Franzen A, et al. Transformation of fetal secondary cartilage into embryonic bone in organ cultures of human mandibular condyles. Cell Tissue Res 1993;271:317–22.

Berraquero R, Palacios J, Gamallo C, et al. Prenatal growth of the human mandibular condylar cartilage. Am J Orthod Dentofacial Orthop 1995;108:194–200.

Cesarani A, Tombolini A, Fagnani E, et al. The anterior ligament of the human malleus. Acta Anat 1991;142:313–6.

Chavez-Lomeli ME, Mansilla Lory J, Pompa JA, Kjaer I. The human mandibular canal arises from three separate canals innervating different tooth groups. J Dent Res 1996;75:1540–4.

Chitty LS, Campbell S, Altman DG. Measurement of the fetal mandible—feasibility and construction of a centile chart. Prenat Diagn 1993;13:749–56.

Czerwinski F, Mahaczek-Kordowska A. Microangiographic studies on vascularization of the human fetal corpus of the mandible. Folia Morphol (Warsz) 1992;51:43–8.

Kjaer I. Formation and early prenatal location of the human mental foramen. Scand J Dent Res 1989;97:1–7.

Kjaer I, Bagheri A. Prenatal development of the alveolar bone of human deciduous incisors and canines. J Dent Res 1999;78:667–72.

Mandarim-de-Lacerda CA, Alves MU. Human mandibular prenatal growth: bivariate and multivariate growth allometry comparing different mandibular dimensions. Anat Embryol 1992;186:537–41.

Merida-Velasco JA, Sanchez-Montesinos I, Espin-Ferra J, et al. Developmental differences in the ossification process of the human corpus and ramus mandibulae. Anat Rec 1993; 235:319–24.

Orliaguet T, Darcha C, Dechelotte P, Vanneuville G. Meckel's cartilage in the human embryo and fetus. Anat Rec 1994;238:491–7.

Orliaguet T, Dechelotte P, Scheye T, Vanneuville G. Relations between Meckel's cartilage and the morphogenesis of the mandible in the human embryo. Surg Radiol Anat 1993;15:41–6.

Orliaguet T, Dechelotte P, Scheye T, Vanneuville G. The relationship between Meckel's cartilage and the development of the human fetal mandible. Surg Radiol Anat 1993;15:113–8.

Ouchi Y, Abe S, Sun-Ki R, et al. Attachment of the sphenomandibular ligament to bone during intrauterine embryo development for the control of mandibular movement. Bull Tokyo Dent Coll 1998;39:91–4.

Rodriguez-Vazquez JF, Merida-Velasco JR, Arraez-Aybar LA, Jimenez-Collado J. A duplicated Meckel's cartilage in a human fetus. Anat Embryol 1997;195:497–502.

Rodriguez-Vazquez JF, Merida-Velasco JR, Jimenez-Collado J. A study of the os goniale in man. Acta Anat 1991;142:188–92.

Rodriguez-Vazquez JF, Merida-Velasco JR, Jimenez-Collado J. Development of the human sphenomandibular ligament. Anat Rec 1992;233:453–60.

Rodriguez-Vazquez JF, Merida-Velasco JR, Merida-Velasco JA, et al. Development of Meckel's cartilage in the symphyseal region in man. Anat Rec 1997;249:249–54.

Sherer DM, Metlay LA, Woods JR Jr. Lack of mandibular movement manifested by absent fetal swallowing: a possible factor in the pathogenesis of micrognathia. Am J Perinatol 1995;12:30–3.

Uchida Y, Akiyoshi T, Goto M, Katsuki T. Morphological changes of human mandibular bone during fetal periods. Okajimas Folia Anat Jpn 1994;71:227–47.

Watson WJ, Katz VL. Sonographic measurement of the fetal mandible: standards for normal pregnancy. Am J Perinatol 1993;10:226–8.

13 TEMPOROMANDIBULAR JOINT

NORMAL DEVELOPMENT

The temporomandibular joint is a secondary development in both evolutionary (phylogenetic) and embryological (ontogenetic) history. The joint between the malleus and incus that develops at the dorsal end of Meckel's cartilage is phylogenetically the primary jaw joint and is homologous with the jaw joint of reptiles. With both evolutionary and embryological development of the middle-ear chamber, this primary Meckel's joint loses its association with the mandible, reflecting the adaption of the bones of the primitive jaw joint to sound conduction (see Chapter 18). The mammalian temporomandibular joint develops as an entirely new and separate jaw-joint mechanism.

In the human fetus, the primitive joint within Meckel's cartilage (before the malleus and incus form) functions briefly as a jaw joint, mouth-opening movements having started at 8 weeks post conception, well before development of the definitive temporomandibular joint. When the temporomandibular joint forms at 10 weeks, both the incudomalleal and definitive jaw joints move in synchrony, for about 8 weeks in fetal life. Both are moved by muscles supplied by the same mandibular division of the trigeminal nerve (ie, the tensor tympani to the malleus and the masticatory muscles to the mandible).

The embryonic development of the temporomandibular joint differs considerably from that of other synovial joints, reflecting its complicated evolutionary history. Most synovial joints complete the development of their initial cavity by the 7th week post conception, but the temporomandibular joint does

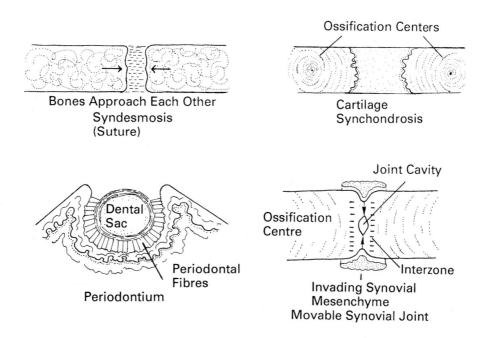

Figure 13–1 Embryonic origins of various types of joints.

not start to appear until this time. Whereas limb joints develop directly into their adult form by cavity formation within the single blastema from which both adjoining endochondral bones develop (Fig. 13–1), the temporomandibular joint develops from initially widely separated temporal and condylar blastemata that grow towards each other (Fig. 13–2). The temporal blastema arises from the otic capsule, a component of the basicranium that forms the petrous temporal bone. The condylar blastema arises from the secondary condylar cartilage of the mandible. In contrast to other synovial joints, fibrous cartilage (rather than hyaline cartilage) forms on the articular facets of the temporal mandibular fossa and mandibular condyle. In the latter site, the underlying secondary cartilage acts as a growth center.

Because Meckel's cartilage plays no part in the development of the mandibular condyle, it does not contribute to the formation of the definitive temporomandibular joint. Membranous bone forming lateral to Meckel's cartilage, first appearing at 6 weeks post conception, forms the initial mandibular body and ramus. Concomitantly, the lateral pterygoid muscle develops medial

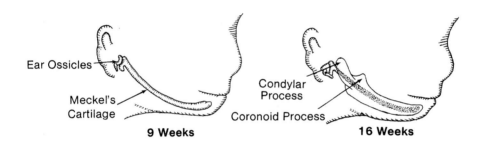

9 Weeks　　　　　　　**16 Weeks**

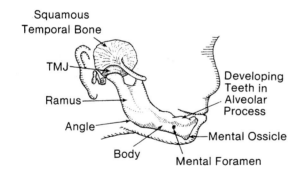

Neonate Mandible

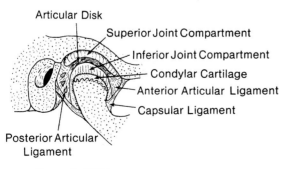

Neonate TMJ

Figure 13–2 Development of the mandible and the temporomandibular joint (TMJ).

to the future condylar area and initiates movement of Meckel's cartilage by its contractions at 8 weeks, functioning through the primary meckelian joint.

Between the 10th and 12th weeks post conception, the accessory mandibular condylar cartilage develops as the first blastema, growing toward the later-developing temporal blastema. The temporal articular fossa is initially convex but progressively assumes its definitive concave shape. The initially wide intervening mesenchyme is narrowed by condylar growth and differentiates into layers of fibrous tissue. During the 10th week, two clefts develop in the interposed vascular fibrous connective tissue, forming the two joint cavities and thereby defining the intervening articular disk. The inferior compartment forms first (at 10 weeks), separating the future disk from the developing condyle, and the upper compartment starts to appear at about 11½ weeks. Cavitation occurs by degradation rather than by enzymic liquefaction or cell death. Synovial-membrane invasion may be necessary for cavitation. Synovial-fluid production by this method lubricates movements in the joint.

Muscle movement is requisite to joint cavitation: the connective tissues separating the initially discrete small spaces have to be ruptured for the spaces to coalesce into functional cavities. Early immobilization of developing joints results in the absence of joint cavities and in fusion of the articulations, with consequent skeletal distortions.

Early functional activity of the temporomandibular joint provides biomechanical stresses that produce ischemia in the differentiating tissues of the joint, facilitating chondrogenesis in the condyle and articular fossa. Functional pressures contribute to the contouring of the articulating surfaces.

The articular disk, appearing at 7½ weeks, is biconcave ab initio, suggesting genetic determination and not functional shaping. It gains thickness and density, subdividing into superior, intermediate, and inferior laminae. The disk is continuous ventrally with the tendon of the lateral pterygoid muscle. The dorsal aspect subdivides its attachments: the superior lamina, following the contour of the squamous temporal bone, inserts in the region of the petrosquamous fissure; the intermediate lamina continues into the middle ear through the petrotympanic fissure, inserting into the malleus and anterior ligament of the malleus (diskomalleolar ligament); and the inferior lamina curves caudally and inserts into the dorsal aspect of the mandibular condyle.

A condensation of mesenchyme forms the anlage of the joint capsule, progressively isolating the joint with its synovial membrane from the surrounding tissues. The joint capsule, composed of fibrous tissue and recognizable by the 11th week post conception, forms lateral ligaments.

The temporomandibular joint of the newborn child is a comparatively lax structure, with stability solely dependent on the capsule surrounding the joint; it is more mobile then than at any time later. At birth, the mandibular fossa is almost flat and bears no articular tubercle. Only after eruption of the permanent dentition at 7 years does the articular tubercle begin to become prominent; its development accelerates until the 12th year of life. When the condyle is absent, there is no well-defined fossa or tubercle.

The joint structures grow laterally, concomitant with the widening of the neurocranium. The temporal element, rather than the condyles, is critical in establishing this lateral growth. The articular surface of the fossa and tubercle becomes more fibrous and less vascular with age. In postnatal life, as the articular tubercle grows, the disk changes shape and becomes more compact, less cellular, and more collagenous. The mature disk is avascular and aneural in its central portion but is filled with vessels, nerves, and elastic fibers posteriorly attaching it to the squamotympanic suture.

ANOMALIES OF DEVELOPMENT

Defective development of the temporomandibular joint results in ankylosis, producing immobilization and impaired mandibular formation. Absence of all elements of the joint is exceedingly rare. Failure of cavitation of one or both joint compartments results in uni- or bilateral ankylosis. The functionless joint results in mandibular maldevelopment, with masticatory distress of varying severity. Whereas absence of the articular disk is exceedingly rare, its perforation (resulting in intercompartmental communication) is fairly common and is not necessarily debilitating.

Selected Bibliography

Ashworth GJ. The attachments of the temporomandibular joint meniscus in the human fetus. Br J Oral Maxillofac Surg 1990;28:246–50.

Bach-Petersen S, Kjaer I, Fischer-Hansen B. Prenatal development of the human osseous temporomandibular region. J Craniofac Genet Dev Biol 1994;14:135–43.

Berraquero R, Palacios J, Gamallo C, et al. Prenatal growth of the human mandibular condylar cartilage. Am J Orthod Dentofacial Orthop 1995;108:194–200.

Merida-Velasco JR, Rodriguez-Vazquez JF, Merida-Velasco JA, et al. Development of the human temporomandibular joint. Anat Rec 1999;255:20–33.

Merida-Velasco JR, Rodriguez-Vazquez JF, Merida-Velasco JA, Jimenez-Collado J. The vascular relationship between the temporomandibular joint and the middle ear in the human fetus. J Oral Maxillofac Surg 1999;57:146–53.

Naidoo LC. The development of the temporomandibular joint: a review with regard to the lateral pterygoid muscle. J Dent Assoc S Africa 1993;48:189–94.

Ogutcen-Toller M. The morphogenesis of the human discomalleolar and sphenomandibular ligaments. J Craniomaxillofac Surg 1995;23:42–6.

Ogutcen-Toller M, Juniper RP. The embryologic development of the human lateral pterygoid muscle and its relationships with the temporomandibular joint disc and Meckel's cartilage. J Oral Maxillofac Surg 1993;51:772–9.

Ogutcen-Toller M, Juniper RP. The development of the human lateral pterygoid muscle and the temporomandibular joint and related structures: a three-dimensional approach. Early Hum Dev 1994;39:57–68.

Radlanski RJ, Lieck S, Bontschev NE. Development of the human temporomandibular joint. Computer-aided 3D-reconstructions. Eur J Oral Sci 1999;107:25–34.

Ramieri G, Bonardi G, Morani V, et al. Development of nerve fibres in the temporomandibular joint of the human fetus. Anat Embryol 1996;194:57–64.

Razook SJ, Gotcher JE Jr, Bays RA. Temporomandibular joint noises in infants: review of the literature and report of cases. Oral Surg Oral Med Oral Pathol 1989;67:658–64.

Robinson PD, Poswillo DE. Temporomandibular joint development in the marmoset—a mirror of man. J Craniofac Genet Dev Biol 1994;14:245–51.

Rodriguez-Vazquez JF, Merida-Velasco JR, Jimenez-Collado J. Relationships between the temporomandibular joint and the middle ear in human fetuses. J Dent Res 1993;72:62–6.

Sato I, Ishikawa H, Shimada K, et al. Morphology and analysis of the development of the human temporomandibular joint and masticatory muscle. Acta Anat 1994;149:55–62.

Valenza V, Farina E, Carini F. The prenatal morphology of the articular disk of the human temporomandibular joint. Ital J Anat Embryol 1993;98:221–30.

14 SKULL GROWTH: SUTURES AND CEPHALOMETRICS

In cranial development, the contents induce the container . . .

J. Schowing, 1974

The hard and unyielding nature of the bones of the skull that are studied post mortem belie the plasticity of bone tissue in the living. It is this plasticity, responsive to the influences of the surrounding soft tissues and the metabolism of the individual, that allows bone growth (and incidentally, bone distortions) to occur.

The mechanisms of bone growth are described in Chapter 6; it is the purpose of the present chapter to collate the growth of all the disparate components of the skull (detailed in Chapters 7 to 13), to provide a basis for clinical analysis of the growing skull. Little attention has been paid to the prenatal *growth* of the skull compared with its prenatal *development*. Further, most studies have focused on postnatal skull growth because of its clinical significance and the possibilities of therapeutic intervention in the event of abnormalities.

Skull growth is studied at both the macro- and microscopic levels. Anatomically, one can calculate changes from measurements of shape, size, and structure of postmortem material and with cephalometric radiographic techniques in the living. Comparison of distances between radiologic landmarks on skull radiographs provides a basis for assessing facial growth patterns. The measurement of distances between landmarks and of the angles between skull planes constitutes cephalometrics, a science employed in diagnostic orthodontics. Microscopically, the examination of bone growth involves studying osteoblastic and osteoclastic activity, studying vascular alterations, and correlating patterns of lamellar organization with surface remodeling. Microradiography reveals the progress of mineralization in bone trabeculae, and labeling with radioactive isotopes and intravital dyes provides information about sites of bone deposition and resorption. Intravital bone-labeling dyes will show the contour of bone growth by three-dimensional reconstruction of serial sections of bone tissue.

Skull growth results from a combination of (1) bone remodeling (deposition and resorption; see p. 71), (2) apposition of bone at sutures and synchondroses, and (3) transposition-displacement of enlarged and remodeled bones.

SYNCHONDROSES

Endochondral-bone junction sites where cartilage is interposed between contiguous bones are known as synchondroses. Skull growth may occur by intrinsic cartilage growth or by endochondral-bone apposition. Most of the synchondroses that exist prenatally disappear soon after birth. The most persistent is the spheno-occipital synchondrosis (see p. 99), of significance in postnatal skull growth. The sphenoethmoidal junction may persist postnatally as a synchondrosis although desmolytic degeneration of the cartilage produces a suture that is of minimal significance in postnatal growth even though fusing occurs only late in adolescence.

The synchondroses within the condylar areas of the occipital bones may contribute slightly to skull growth; they start to fuse between 3 and 4 years of age (see p. 94). The three synchondroses between the four parts of the prenatal sphenoid bone (the midsphenoidal synchondrosis between the presphenoid and postsphenoid, and the bilateral synchondroses between the body and greater wings of the sphenoid) fuse at birth and thus do not contribute to postnatal skull growth.

SUTURES

Sutures are one of a variety of immovable bone joints (synarthroses) that by definition are limited to the skull. Their locations are genetically determined, but environmental stresses influence their forms. Sutures play a significant role in skull growth. Although they form a firm bond between adjacent bones, they allow slight movement and thus absorb mechanical stress. Intramembranous skull bones are separated by a zone of connective tissue (the sutural ligament or membrane) made up of several layers (Fig. 14–1). The sutural ligament is part of the initial membrane in which the bones ossify. The suture sites appear to inhibit osteogenesis by a cellular degeneration mechanism (apoptosis) that differs from necrosis in that the cells participate in this process, which determines the site's location between encroaching adjacent bones. The sutures of the calvaria differ from those of the facial skeleton, reflecting the slightly different mechanisms of intramembranous osteogenesis in the two areas. The calvarial bones develop in the ectomeninx, and their intervening sutures are composed of parallel fibers continuous with the pericranium and dura mater. By contrast, the facial bones ossify in relatively

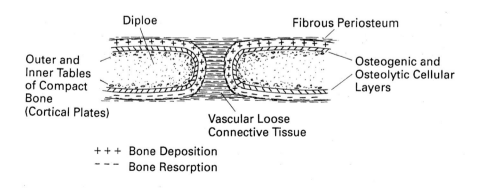

Figure 14–1 Schematic diagram of suture between calvarial bones.

unstructured mesenchyme, each forming a separate periosteal fibrous covering whose fibers are tangential to the bone, with no fibers uniting adjacent bones until a sutural junction is near. Secondary cartilage is a component of some sutures, predominantly in the sagittal and midpalatal sutures. As it also appears in fracture-healing sites, this intramembranous cartilage may indicate mechanical stress. The possible contribution of sutural cartilages to skull growth has not been assessed.

The skull contains the following types of suture:

1. Serrate. The bone edges are sawlike or notched. Examples are the sagittal and coronal sutures; together with the convex shape of the articulating parietal and frontal bones, these sutures enable the cranium to withstand blows of considerable force.
2. Denticulate. The small toothlike projections of the articulating bones widen toward their free ends. This union provides an even more effective interlocking than does a serrate suture. An example is the lambdoid suture.
3. Squamous or beveled. One bone overlaps another, as at the squamous suture between the temporal and parietal bones. The articulating bones are reciprocally beveled, one internally, one externally. The beveled surfaces may be mutually ridged or serrated.
4. Plane or butt-end. The flat-end contiguous bone surfaces are usually roughened and irregular in a complementary manner. An example is the midpalatal suture.

Other types of fibrous joints in the skull are more specialized and are not classified as sutures. Schindylesis is a "tongue-and-groove" type of articulation in which the thin plate of one bone fits into a cleft in another. An example is the articulation of the perpendicular plate of the ethmoid bone with the vomer. Gomphosis is a "peg-in-hole" type of articulation in which a conical process of

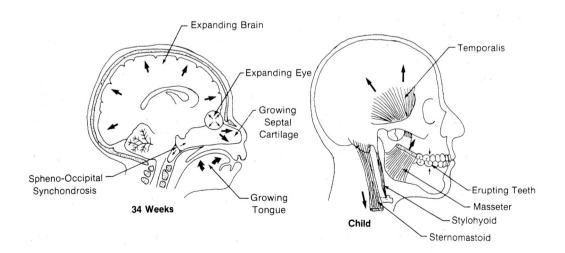

Figure 14–2 Functional matrices operating on skull growth.

one bone is inserted into a socketlike portion of another. An example is the initial (prefusion) styloid process articulation with the petrous temporal bone. By extension, the attachments of teeth into the dental alveoli of the maxilla and mandible are described as gomphoses. The coronal and sagittal sutures, by interdigitation of the projections from the frontal and parietal bones, assume a multigomphosis joint structure to resist mechanical forces exerted at the sutures.

Growth at Suture Sites

Sutures are the sites of cellular proliferation and fiber formation where appositional osteogenesis contributes to growth of the adjacent bones. Experimental evidence indicates that sutural bone growth compensates for the separating forces that are the primary determinants of skull growth. Bone separation is not a pure translatory movement but rather an alternating oscillatory movement. It responds to functional matrices operating by pressure or tension on the bones arising from organ growth or muscle pull (Fig. 14–2).

Changes in head shape are also subject to external factors such as molding at birth, abnormal pressures, and increasing nasopharyngeal capacity with increasing body size (Fig. 14–3).

(For further discussion of this topic, see p. 73 and p. 85.)

Sutural Fusion

Closure or fusion of sutures by intramembranous ossification converts syndesmoses into synostoses. Such fusion effectively closes off further growth potential at a suture site. Sutures begin to fuse on both the outer and inner tables of skull bones simultaneously, but closure on the outer table is slower, more variable, and less complete. There is great variation in the timing of sutural closures, making this phenomenon an unreliable criterion of age. However, some sutures consistently close before others.

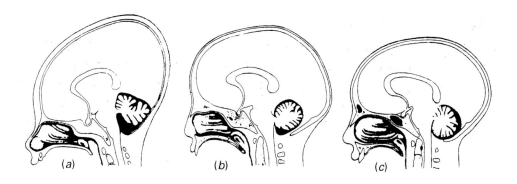

Figure 14–3 Changes in skull and nasopharyngeal shape in sagittal sections of (a) a neonate, (b) a 6-year-old, and (c) a 13-year-old. Note the distended neurocranium at birth and the enlarging nasopharyngeal capacity with increasing age. (Not drawn to scale)

The interfrontal or metopic suture starts closing after the 1st year and is usually obliterated by 7 years of age, thereby converting the paired frontal bones into a single bone. (Persistence of the metopic suture into adulthood occurs in approximately 15 percent of individuals.) The sagittal, coronal, and lambdoidal sutures fuse between 20 and 40 years of age. The occipitomastoid, sphenotemporal, and squamous sutures may not be completely fused even at 70 years of age.

Craniosynostosis

Premature fusion of sutures (synostosis) results in the premature cessation of sutural growth. Abnormal intrauterine compression of the cranium is a factor in causing premature fusion because it alters the immature sutural tissue and initiates mineralization of the sutural ligament. Synostosis is largely confined to the calvaria. It is far less common in the face because of early structural differences in facial and calvarial sutures: the former are composed of periosteal capsules whereas the latter are layered in the directions of bone growth.

Continued bone growth occurs at right angles to the fused suture, with consequent abnormal compensatory growth in other directions that results in distortions of skull shape. The effects of premature synostosis on skull shape depend on the location of the sutures and on the timing of the fusion, and may be part of certain malformation syndromes (eg, Apert syndrome [acrocephalosyndactyly] and Crouzon syndrome [craniofacial dysostosis]).

Suture closure is also sensitive to brain growth; for example, sutures and fontanelles close prematurely in microcephaly, and fusion of sutures is delayed in hydrocephaly.

Isolated premature synostoses produce characteristic skull distortions as a result of redirected continued neural growth toward the patent sutures. Synostosis of the sagittal suture limits lateral skull growth, redirecting growth anteroposteriorly. Bilateral synostosis of the coronal sutures limits the anteroposterior growth of the calvaria, producing a pointed (oxycephaly) or short (brachycephaly) skull; premature synostosis of one side of the coronal or lambdoidal suture causes obliquity of the skull (plagiocephaly). The degree of skull deformity depends upon the number of sutures involved and the time of onset of the premature fusion (the earlier the synostosis, the greater the deformity).

Premature fusion of the synchondroses of the skull base causes underdevelopment of the middle third of the face (see p. 96), with a reduced cranial base, excessive vaulting of the calvaria, and (in some cases) anomalies such as exophthalmia, midfacial hypoplasia, and dental malocclusion.

CRANIOFACIAL GROWTH

The rapid directional growth of the basicranial cartilages and Meckel's cartilage between 7 and 10 weeks post conception accounts for the typical facial changes and appearances before ossification. Because growth movements of the cartilages are important to the spatial relocation of the developing facial bones, alterations in cartilage growth at this time may have significant irreversible consequences for later craniofacial morphology.

Craniofacial growth patterns may be subdivided into three components. The first and general component—accounting for most variation—is allometric, defining variations in proportions related to size increase. Factors residual to and independent of size discriminate shape. Brain growth predominates in the fetal period, flattening the cranial base. This base determines the displacement of the nasomaxillary segment; growth of the orbital contents and nasal septum becomes less important as their relative sizes decrease. The period of greatest displacement of the nasomaxillary segment (downward and forward "growth") is between the 2nd and 3rd months post conception, concomitant with precocious expansion of the temporal lobes of the cerebrum. In anencephaly, the absence of the brain results in the cranial base remaining unflattened, allowing the facial bones to occupy anomalous positions. During the 2nd and 3rd months, the mandible first lags behind the maxilla in growth and then speeds up to regain parity.

The second component of regional variation is alveolar remodeling. Alveolar development and growth is entirely dependent on the presence of tooth buds or teeth. In their absence, no alveolar bone develops, diminishing the height of the facial skeleton. The third component is mandibular condylar growth. As a result of accumulating differences in size and related proportional changes in shape, sexual dimorphism progressively favors males over females as both age. Timing of the condylar growth spurt, as evident from the ramus height, produces secondary dimorphism that diminishes after adolescence.

After 4 years of age, craniofacial growth is not proportional. Neurocranial components grow relatively the least, and mandibular parts grow the most; the other facial components have intermediate patterns of relative growth.

CEPHALOMETRICS

Orthodontists use cephalometrics routinely as a treatment-planning aid. Different cephalographic images are frequently requested; they include the traditional lateral cephalogram, variants such as the 45° oblique and corrected oblique cephalograms, and the posteroanterior cephalogram, used mostly to study asymmetries of the frontal view of the craniofacial region. Growth data from 6 to 20 years for males and females are available at centers such as the Burlington Growth Center at the University of Toronto, and serial cephalometric images noted provide valuable information on the growth and development of the craniofacial environment (Fig. 14–4). Cephalometrics developed as a result of measurements made by anthropologists using craniometric measurements of skulls stabilized in a craniostat. Cephalometrics literally means "measuring the head" as translated from the Greek words *kaphalokis* and *metron*. The development of the cephalostat in the early 1930s resulted in cephalometrics becoming not only popular as a clinical tool but also valuable as a method for studying growth and development changes.

Few (if any) of the areas, points, and planes that orthodontists and anthropologists use as fixed landmarks are stationary. Implanted metallic markers move during growth by shifting with the surface to which they are attached, by being covered with new bone, or (conversely) by being exposed by resorption and then freed from their site. Bone-growth markers such as metal implants, intravital staining, or radioisotope labels give information about static areas for limited periods only during active growth.

Prediction of Growth Patterns

Statistical analysis of serial radiographic measurements by computers provides a new tool for determining skull growth. Calculations of mean growth patterns for large defined populations establish standards that enable one to predict statistically the probable growth patterns of individual children in that population. Prediction of the craniofacial growth pattern (in particular, the growth direction of the maxilla and mandible) will assist the clinician in treatment planning. Extreme deviations from the average, however, result in more difficult, if not impossible, prediction. Researchers have thus investigated numerous parameters (morphologic and radiologic) in an attempt to minimize this problem and to aid the clinician in setting treatment goals. These serial morphologic and cephalometric parameters assist in prediction. Physical change measurements include postural height changes, body weight changes, and physiologic changes, especially during adolescence. Cephalometric measurements, which show correlation with growth and development changes, include frontal sinus size, cranial base deflection, porion position, facial axis changes (Y axis, or mandibular growth axis), molar relationship, mandibular and maxillary length differences, mandibular symphysis morphology (long and thin versus short and wide), condylar length and deflection, face-to-height ratios, ramus deflection, and interincisal angulation. The visual treatment objective (VTO) is a cephalometric tool that became popular in the '70s and '80s. It is often mistaken for a growth prediction protocol; however, it was developed mostly to assist in short-term treatment planning. The average orthodontic treatment during adolescence lasts approximately 2 years, and a fairly accurate prediction is possible during this short period. Long-term prediction methods have been described, but they have had limited success. It was recommended that the VTO be used to set visual treatment goals, which could include the predicted dental, skeletal, and soft-tissue objectives. Obviously, this visual picture is a tremendous teaching tool. During the '90s, aesthetics reigned supreme, and such prediction and setting of visual goals aided in the attainment of an ideal soft-tissue profile. Clinical studies have shown that few clinicians venture into the field of visual treatment goal setting, mainly because of the complexity of the craniofacial growth process and the difficulty in manually preparing a VTO. However, there has been an explosion in computerization in dentistry. Most computer-generated cephalometric analyses include a VTO or treatment prediction function (Fig. 14–5). The ease of contemporary computer use could revitalize the use of prediction schemes for short- and long-term craniofacial changes.

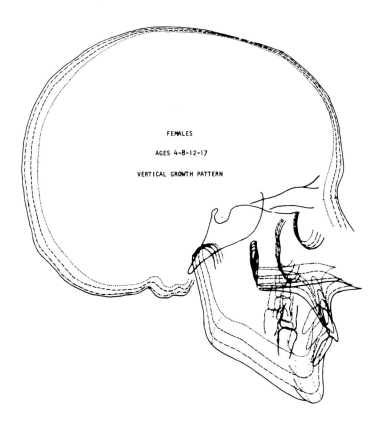

Figure 14–4 Superimpositions of a vertical growth pattern depicted form 4 to 17 years. Growth of the face can occur in a vertical, average, and horizontal direction.

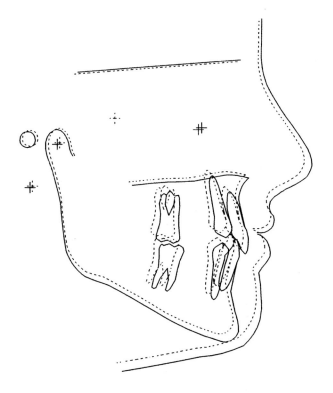

Figure 14–5 Example of a growth estimate or visual treatment objective using the pretreatment cephalometric tracing as a basis to show possible growth changes over 2 years of orthodontic treatment.

Interceptive therapy might be undertaken on the basis of the prediction, to minimize undesirable facial and dental growth patterns. Interceptive therapy is an important phase of orthodontic treatment and is used mostly during the early to late mixed-dentition stage. A VTO uses aspects of normal growth and development, such as the development of the dentition from the primary through the mixed to a normal occlusion. To provide a visual picture of the predicted changes, tooth size/arch size space discrepancies as well as subsequent cephalometric incisor correction need to be incorporated into the analysis.

CRANIOFACIAL ANALYSIS

Radiographic cephalometry is now widely used clinically for analysis of craniofacial forms, and cephalometric parameters provide information regarding aspects such as facial typing, profile types, growth directions, and general classification of malocclusions. Cephalometrics are applied periodically on growing children; this provides longitudinal growth measurements (see Fig. 14–4). Moreover, the superimposition of pre- and post-treatment cephalometric tracings and the comparison of cephalometric measurements also ensure that treatment objectives are met. It thus serves as a form of quality control for treatment rendered. Standardized positioning of the head in cephalostats is imperative to allow the superimposition of serial lateral and frontal skull radiographs of an individual for the calculation of growth data. Standardized radiologic landmarks and artificial planes and angles are used for cephalometric analyses; because growth changes render them unstable, great care should be exercised in their use in analysis. The availability of cephalometric data from growth centers enables the clinician and researcher alike to compare normal cephalometric parameters to those values provided by cephalometric analyses of malocclusions or aberrant growth patterns.

The principal radiologic landmarks (Fig. 14–6) and their clinically recognized abbreviations are as follows:

1. Nasion (N), the most depressed point of the frontonasal suture
2. Anterior nasal spine (ANS), the most anterior point of the nasal cavity floor
3. Subspinale (point A), the most depressed point on the concavity between the anterior nasal spine and prosthion
4. Prosthion (P), the most anterior point of the maxillary alveolus
5. Infradentale (I), the most anterior point of the mandibular alveolus
6. Supramentale (point B), the most depressed point on the concavity between infradentale and pogonion
7. Pogonion (Pg), the most anterior point of the bony chin
8. Gnathion (Gn), the point where the anterior and lower borders of the mandible meet
9. Menton (M), the lowest point of the mandible
10. Gonion (Go), the point of intersection of the mandibular base line and posterior ramus line

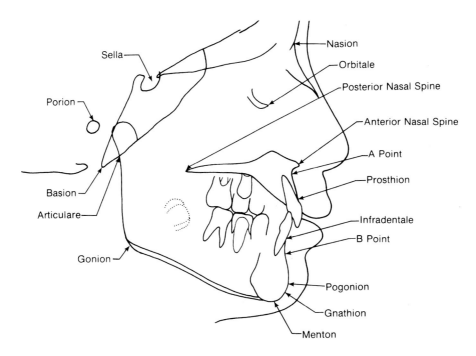

Figure 14–6 Cephalometric tracing of a lateral-view radiograph of a 12-year-old child, depicting the radiologic landmarks used in cephalometrics. (Courtesy of Dr. K. E. Glover)

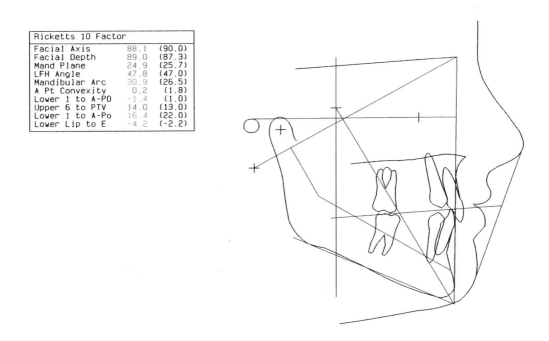

Ricketts 10 Factor		
Facial Axis	88.1	(90.0)
Facial Depth	89.0	(87.3)
Mand Plane	24.9	(25.7)
LFH Angle	47.8	(47.0)
Mandibular Arc	30.9	(26.5)
A Pt Convexity	0.2	(1.8)
Lower 1 to A-PO	-1.4	(1.0)
Upper 6 to PTV	14.0	(13.0)
Lower 1 to A-Po	16.4	(22.0)
Lower Lip to E	-4.2	(-2.2)

Figure 14–7 In contemporary orthodontics, various cephalometric analyses exist that provide a description of facial form; the Ricketts analysis is such an example. Normal values of the measured parameters exist for age, gender, and race for a specific subject. Normal values are shown in parentheses.

11. Articulare (Ar), the point of intersection of the inferior cranial base and the posterior surface of the mandibular condyles
12. Sella (S), the midpoint of the sella turcica (pituitary fossa)
13. Basion (Ba), the midpoint on the anterior margin of the foramen magnum (the posterior end of the midline cranial base)
14. Orbitale (O), the lowest point of the inferior border of the orbital cavity
15. Posterior nasal spine (PNS), the most posterior midline point of the hard palate
16. Porion (Po), the midpoint of the upper margin of the external acoustic meatus
17. Bolton point (BP), the highest point of the curve between the occipital condyle and the lower border of the occipital bone
18. Registration point (R), the midpoint of the perpendicular from sella to the Bolton-nasion line

The chief radiologic planes are as follows:

- Frankfort plane, the line passing through porion and orbitale
- Sella-nasion plane, the line passing through sella and nasion (SN)
- Occlusal plane, the line passing through the occlusal surfaces of the posterior teeth
- Mandibular plane, the line tangent to the lower border of the mandible passing through menton
- Palatal plane, the line joining anterior and posterior nasal spines
- Facial plane, the vertical line joining nasion to pogonion
- Bolton plane, the line from Bolton point to nasion
- Y axis (growth axis), the line from sella to gnathion

Various cephalometric analyses are available for the clinical evaluation of facial form of which the Steiner and Ricketts analyses are prime examples (Fig. 14–7); the clinician can select the linear and angular measurements and/or interrelationships thought to provide the best assessment of the individual patient's facial disproportion. In most cases, the relationship of the various measurements, lines, planes, and angles is more important than the absolute value of a specific measurement. The distinction between cephalometric hard- and soft-tissue images initiated many efforts to provide ideal images for analysis and study purposes. Often, a compromise had to be accepted between hard- and soft-tissue clarity. Techniques such as xeroradiography (used for mammography) found their way into orthodontics. However, the latter quickly disappeared due to high radiation and expense. Mechanical refinement of the cephalostat, screens, filters, and films soon provided superb images.

Three-dimensional optical laser scanning techniques have been introduced into the field of growth and development. The use of scanning methods is only in its infancy, and indications are already apparent for use in the study of facial changes during treatment, especially during facial reconstruction, and in forensic science. Optical scanners are also being miniaturized, and portable scanners are already in use by criminologists and the military. Optical scanning, which can provide enhanced three-dimensional scanned images, provides a new medium whereby facial characteristics can be studied. In the future, use of this scanning tool may assist the conversion of the data presently housed in Growth Centers such as the Burlington Growth Center at the University of Toronto.

As previously noted, data derived from two- and three-dimensional longitudinal growth studies are being used in attempts to develop methods that predict growth more accurately. This will eventually benefit the clinician, who analyzes facial form at the time of examination but who needs to extrapolate to predict how the face will look at a later date with or without treatment.

Selected Bibliography

Andrews LF. The six keys to normal occlusion. Am J Orthod 1972;62:296–309.

Angle EH. Classification of malocclusion. Dent Cosmos 1899;41:246–8,350–70.

Bettega G, Chenin M, Sadek H, et al. Three-dimensional fetal cephalometry. Cleft Palate Craniofac J 1996;33:463–7.

Chadduck WM, Boop FA, Blankenship JB, Husain M. Teningioma and sagittal craniosynostosis in an infant: case report. Neurosurg 1992;30:441–2.

Cohen MM Jr, MacLean RE, editors. Craniosynostosis: diagnosis, evaluation, and management. 2nd ed. Oxford: Oxford University Press; 2000.

Holdaway RA. A soft-tissue cephalometric analysis and its use in orthodontic treatment planning. Part II. Am J Orthod 1984;85:279–93.

Johnson NA. Xeroradiography for cephalometric analysis. Am J Orthod 1976;69:524–6.

Kreiborg S, Cohen MM Jr. Characteristics of the infant Apert skull and its subsequent development. J Craniofac Genet Dev Biol 1990;10:399–410.

Machin GA. Thanatophoric dysplasia in monozygotic twins discordant for cloverleaf skull: prenatal diagnosis, clinical and pathological findings [letter]. Am J Med Genet 1992;44:842–3.

Mathijssen IM, Vaandrager JM, van der Meulen JC, et al. The role of bone centers in the pathogenesis of craniosynostosis: an embryologic approach using CT measurements in isolated craniosynostosis and Apert and Crouzon syndromes. Plast Reconstr Surg 1996;98:17–26.

Mathijssen IM, van Splunder J, Vermeij-Keers C, et al. Tracing craniosynostosis to its developmental stage through bone center displacement. J Craniofac Genet Dev Biol 1999;19:57–63.

Opperman LA, Nolen AA, Ogle RC. TGF-beta 1, TGF-beta 2, and TGF-beta 3 exhibit distinct patterns of expression during cranial suture formation and obliteration in vivo and in vitro. J Bone Miner Res 1997;12:301–10.

Opperman LA, Passarelli RW, Morgan EP, et al. Cranial sutures require tissue interactions with dura mater to resist osseous obliteration in vitro. J Bone Miner Res 1995;10:1978–87.

Popovich F, Thompson GW. Craniofacial templates for orthodontic case analysis. In: Hardin JW, editor. Clark's clinical dentistry. Philadelphia: J.B. Lippincott Company; 1976. p. 1–15.

Pretorius DH, Nelson TR. Prenatal visualization of cranial sutures and fontanelles with three-dimensional ultrasonography. J Ultrasound Med 1994;13:871–6.

Ricketts RM, Bench RW, Gugino CF, et al. Bioprogressive theraphy. Book 1. Denver: Rocky Mountain Orthodontics; 1979. p. 35–69.

Steiner CC. Cephalometric in clinical practice. Angle Orthod 1959;29:8–29.

Stelnicki EJ, Vanderwall K, Harrison MR, et al. The in utero correction of unilateral coronal craniosynostosis. Plast Reconstr Surg 1997;101:262–9.

15 TONGUE AND TONSILS

THE TONGUE

Normal Development

The tongue arises in the ventral wall of the primitive oropharynx from the inner lining of the first four pharyngeal arches. The covering oropharyngeal mucous membrane rises into the developing mouth as a swelling sac, the result of invasion by muscle tissue from the occipital somites.

During the 4th week post conception, paired lateral thickenings of mesenchyme appear on the internal aspect of the first pharyngeal arches to form the lingual swellings (Fig. 15–1). Between and behind these swellings, a median eminence appears, the tuberculum impar (unpaired tubercle), whose caudal border is marked by a blind pit. This pit, the foramen caecum, marks the site of origin of the thyroid diverticulum, an endodermal duct that appears during the somite period. The diverticulum migrates caudally ventral to the pharynx (Fig. 15–2) as the thyroglossal duct, which bifurcates and subdivides to form the thyroid gland. Thyroid tissue occasionally remains in the substance of the tongue, giving rise to a lingual thyroid gland. The gland descends to reach its definitive level caudal to the thyroid cartilage at the end of the 7th week. The thyroglossal duct normally disintegrates and disappears between the 5th and 10th weeks. The caudal attachment of the duct may persist as the pyramidal lobe of the thyroid gland.

The lingual swellings grow and fuse with each other, encompassing the tuberculum impar, to provide the ectodermally derived mucosa of the body

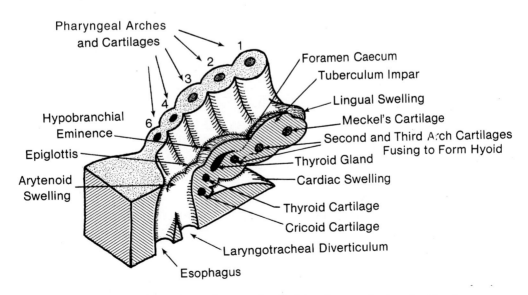

Figure 15–1 Tongue primordia arising in the ventral wall of the pharynx of a 4-week-old embryo.

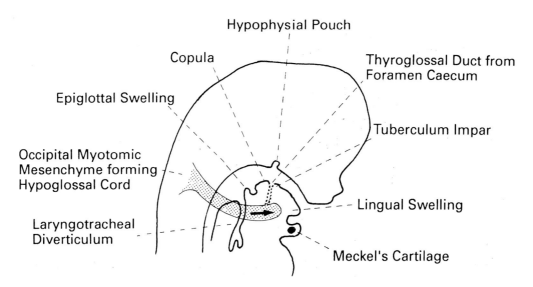

Figure 15–2 Schematic paramedian section of a 5-week-old embryo, illustrating development of the ventral wall of the oropharynx and the path of migration of the occipital-somite myotomes forming the tongue muscles.

(anterior two-thirds) of the tongue (Fig. 15–3).* Around the periphery of the fused and elevated lingual swellings, there is an epithelial proliferation into the underlying mesenchyme. Degeneration of the central cells of this horseshoe-shaped lamina forms a sulcus (the linguogingival groove), which frees the body of the tongue from the floor of the mouth except for the midline frenulum of the tongue.

The ventral bases of the second, third, and fourth pharyngeal arches elevate into a single midventral prominence known as the copula. A posterior subdivision of this prominence is identified as the *hypobranchial eminence*. The endodermally derived mucosa of the second to fourth pharyngeal arches and the copula provide the covering for the root (posterior third) of the tongue (Fig. 15–4). The V-shaped sulcus terminalis, whose apex is the foramen caecum, demarcates the mobile body of the tongue from its fixed root (Fig. 15–5). The line of the sulcus terminalis is marked by 8 to 12 large circumvallate papillae that develop at 2 to 5 months post conception. The mucosa of the dorsal surface of the body of the tongue develops fungiform papillae much earlier, at 11 weeks post conception. Filiform papillae develop later and are not complete until after birth. At birth, the root mucosa becomes pitted by deep crypts that develop into the lingual tonsil, the completion of which is marked by lymphocytic infiltration (see Fig. 15–5).

Taste buds arise by inductive interaction between epithelial cells (both ecto- and endodermal) and invading gustatory nerve cells from the chorda tympani (facial), glossopharyngeal, and vagus nerves. Taste buds form in great-

---

*In the adult tongue, it is difficult to identify where the embryonic oropharyngeal membrane demarcated the transition from ectoderm to endoderm. The greater part of the mucosa of the body of the tongue is believed to be of ectodermal origin.

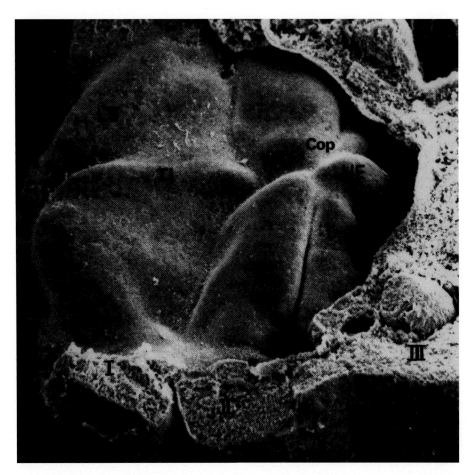

Figure 15–3 Scanning electron micrograph of the developing tongue of a 33- to 35-day-old embryo. The pharyngeal arches (I, II, III) border the floor of the mouth. The lingual swelling (LS) develops from the first pharyngeal arch, the tuberculum impar (TI) between the first and second pharyngeal arches, and the hypobranchial eminence (HE) from the third pharyngeal arch. The foramen caecum (FC) is hidden between the tuberculum impar and the copula (Cop). (× 20 original magnification) (Reproduced with permission from Waterman RE, Meller SM. Prenatal development of the oral cavity and paraoral structures in man. In: Shaw, Sweeney, et al, editors. Textbook of oral biology. Philadelphia: W.B. Saunders Co.; 1978.)

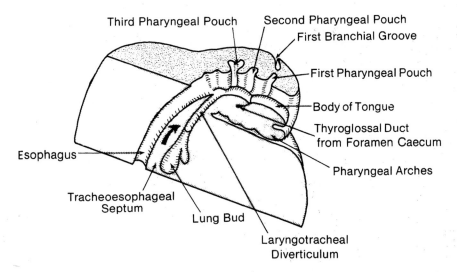

Figure 15–4 Tongue and laryngeal development in a 7-week-old embryo.

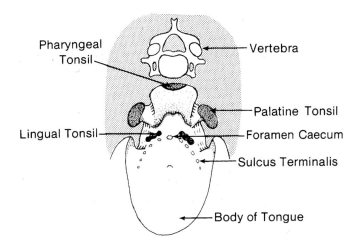

Figure 15–5 Tongue and pharynx of an adult. Note the "ring" of lymphoid tissue formed by the lingual, palatine, and pharyngeal tonsils.

est concentration on the dorsal surface of the tongue and in lesser numbers on the palatoglossal arches, palate, posterior surface of the epiglottis, and posterior wall of the oropharynx. Gustatory cells start to form as early as the 7th week post conception, but taste buds are not recognizable until 13 to 15 weeks, when taste perception is initiated.* Initially, only single taste buds are present in the fungiform papillae, but these multiply in later fetal life, possibly by branching. All of the taste buds in the fungiform papillae of the tongue are present at birth, but some circumvallate taste buds develop postnatally.

The muscles of the tongue arise in the floor of the pharynx in the occipital somite region opposite the origin of the hypoglossal nerve. The muscle mass pushes forward as the hypoglossal cord beneath the mucous layer of the tongue, carrying the hypoglossal nerve along with it. The path of the hypoglossal nerve in the adult is explained by its embryological origins from its dorsally located brain stem origin, tracking ventrally and superficial to the main arteries and nerves and ending under the tongue (see Fig. 15–2).

Diverse embryological sources of the tongue are reflected in its complex innervation. The embryological components of the tongue, while moving upward and ventrally into the mouth, retain their initially established nerve supplies. Thus, the mucosal contributions of the first pharyngeal arch (trigeminal nerve) are reflected in the lingual nerve's tactile sensory supply to the body of the tongue. The second pharyngeal arch (facial nerve) accounts for gustatory sensation from the body of the tongue through the chorda tympani nerve (considered to be a pretrematic branch of the facial nerve that invades first-arch territory). The contributions of the third and fourth arches are recognizable by the mixed tactile and gustatory glossopharyngeal and vagal nerve innervation of the mucosa of the root of the tongue. The palatoglossus muscle is innervated by the pharyngeal plexus, the fibers of which are derived from

---

*In utero taste perception can be used therapeutically to reduce excess amniotic fluid (hydramnios) by the addition of saccharin to the fluid, inducing increased swallowing that reduces the fluid (see footnote, p. 178).

the third and fourth arches (glossopharyngeal and vagus) and accessory nerves. Finally, the motor innervation of all the musculature of the tongue (except the palatoglossus) by the hypoglossal nerve reflects its occipital somite origin.

The tongue's rapid enlargement relative to the space in which it develops results in its occupation of the whole of the stomodeal chamber that will later divide into the mouth, the oropharynx, and the nasopharynx. The initial partition of the stomodeal chamber by the laterally developing palatal shelves is delayed by the relatively enormous tongue reaching from the floor to the roof of the stomodeum. Only with later enlargement of the stomodeum does the tongue descend into the mouth chamber proper, allowing the palatal shelves to close off the mouth from the nasal fossae (see p. 42).

The entire tongue is within the mouth at birth; its posterior third descends into the pharynx by the age of 4 years. The tongue normally doubles in length, breadth, and thickness between birth and adolescence, reaching nearly maximal size by about 8 years of age but continuing to grow in some individuals during adulthood. Its early growth tends to be precocious relative to the size of the mouth, reflecting its early role in suckling. Also, the large tongue in a small mouth partly accounts for the peculiar tongue-thrusting character of the infant's early swallowing pattern, in which the tongue fills the space between the separated jaws during swallowing. The later enlargement of the mouth facilitates the conversion to the adult pattern of swallowing, in which the tip of the tongue lies against the palate behind the maxillary incisor teeth (see p. 180).

The hypobranchial eminence, derived from the bases of the third and fourth pharyngeal arches, forms the epiglottis, which guards the entrance to the larynx during swallowing. Cartilage differentiates within the epiglottis by the 15th week post conception. The epiglottis is well developed by the 21st week and is in full contact with the soft palate by the 23rd to the 25th week. This contact may relate to infant respiratory viability, which enables neonates to breath while swallowing liquids during suckling.

The sites of the second and third pharyngeal arches in the adult pharynx are marked respectively by the anterior and posterior pillars of the fauces, between which the palatine (faucial) tonsils develop. Growth of the third and fourth pharyngeal arches, in contributing to the root of the tongue, obliterates the ventral portions of the first and second pharyngeal pouches, leaving the dorsal portions to develop into the auditory tubes and palatine tonsillar fossae, respectively (see p. 63).

ANOMALIES OF DEVELOPMENT

The retention of an abnormally short lingual frenum results in ankyloglossia (tongue-tie), a fairly common developmental anomaly. Persistence of the thyroglossal duct may give rise to islands of aberrant thyroid tissue, cysts, fistulae, or sinuses in the midline. A lingual thyroid gland at the site of the foramen caecum at the junction of the body and root of the tongue is not uncommon. Because the tongue influences the paths of eruption of the teeth, the state of its development is of considerable interest to the orthodontist.

The tongue may fail to achieve a normal growth rate, resulting in an abnormally small tongue (microglossia) or in overdevelopment (macroglossia). Rarely, the tongue fails to develop (aglossia), or it becomes forked, bifid, or trifid as a result of the failure of its components to fuse. Such clefts are part of the syndrome of orodigitofacial dysostosis, which also manifests as hyperplasia of the labial frenula and as cleft palate. Microglossia characterizes hypodactylia and occurs in persons with cleft palate. Macroglossia typifies anencephaly; trisomy 21 syndrome; Crouzon syndrome; and the association of coloboma of the eye, heart anomaly, choanal atresia, retardation, and genital and ear anomalies (CHARGE syndrome).

THE TONSILS

The endoderm lining the second pharyngeal pouch between the tongue and soft palate invades the surrounding mesenchyme as a group of solid buds. The central parts of these buds degenerate, forming the tonsillar crypts. Invading lymphoid cells surround the crypts, becoming grouped as lymphoid follicles.

Lymphoid tissue invades the palatine, posterior pharyngeal (adenoids), and lingual tonsillar regions in the 3rd to 5th months post conception. These lymphoid masses encircle the oropharynx to form a ring (*Waldeyer's ring*) of immunodefensive tissue that grows markedly postnatally to bulge into the oropharynx (see Fig. 15–5).

The palatine tonsils arise at the site of the second pharyngeal pouch while the pharyngeal and lingual tonsils develop respectively in the mucosa of the posterior wall of the pharynx and in the root of the tongue. Lateral extensions of the lymphoid tissue posterior to the openings of the auditory tubes form the tubal tonsils.

These disparate embryonic origins of the tonsils are reflected in differences in the characteristics of the cytology, growth, and involution of the tonsils. The tonsils are the site of migration of both B and T lymphocytes that synthesize immunoglobulins. Tonsillar growth is variable and cannot be considered true growth but rather the response of each tonsil to the development of immunocompetence. Accordingly, the lymphoid tissue in the four tonsillar sites may not coincide in their growth and regression rates, each achieving its greatest size at a different age and each enlarging individually in response to immunologic challenges. The sizes of the tonsils are thus variable and reflect more the state of tonsillar immunodefence mechanisms than the person's age.

Lymphoid tissue grows faster on the posterior nasopharyngeal wall than elsewhere, achieving its greatest size there by 5 years of age; it thereby narrows the nasopharyngeal airway at this age, with possible consequences for mouth breathing. Thereafter, lymphoid tissue diminishes until the age of 10 years, when it again briefly increases slightly, and then resumes declining in size. The nasopharynx normally enlarges in pre- and early adolescence due to the concurrent accelerated growth of the bony nasopharynx and the involution of the pharyngeal tonsil. Nasopharyngeal enlargement coincides with the adolescent growth spurt to meet increased metabolic demands for oxygen.

The period between 8 and 12 years of age is critical for the eruption of permanent teeth. Muscle imbalances caused by mouth breathing and the infantile pattern of swallowing can adversely influence tooth eruption patterns and facial development. Dental malocclusion and a narrow adenoid facies have been attributed to mouth-breathing habits induced by exuberant pharyngeal ("adenoids") and palatine tonsillar growth. Chronic allergies resulting in pharyngeal mucosal hypertrophy, nasal infections, and mechanical blockage by the conchae or deviation of the nasal septum may also lead to mouth breathing, inducing a syndrome of respiratory obstruction characterized by a tongue-thrusting swallow and dental malocclusion.

Selected Bibliography

Achiron R, Ben Arie A, Gabbay U, et al. Development of the fetal tongue between 14 and 26 weeks of gestation: in utero ultrasonographic measurements. Ultrasound Obstet Gynecol 1997; 9:39–41.

Barlow LA, Northcutt RG. Analysis of the embryonic lineage of vertebrate taste buds. Chem Senses 1994;19:715–24.

Choi G, Suh YL, Lee HM, et al. Prenatal and postnatal changes of the human tonsillar crypt epithelium. Acta Otolaryngol Suppl 1996;523:28–33.

Emmanouil-Nikoloussi EN, Kerameos-Foroglou C. Developmental malformations of human tongue and associated syndromes [review]. Bull Group Int Rech Sci Stomatol Odontol 1992;35:5–12.

Holibka V. High endothelial venules in the developing human palatine tonsil. Adv Otorhinolaryngol 1992;47:54–8.

Kimes KR, Mooney MP, Siegel MI, Todhunter JS. Size and growth rate of the tongue in normal and cleft lip and palate human fetal specimens. Cleft Palate Craniofac J 1991;28:212–6.

Mistretta CM. The role of innervation in induction and differentiation of taste organs: introduction and background. Ann N Y Acad Sci 1998;855:1–13.

Oakley B. Taste neurons have multiple inductive roles in mammalian gustatory development. Ann N Y Acad Sci 1998;855:50–7.

Slipka J. The development and involution of tonsils. Adv Otorhinolaryngol 1992:47:1–4.

Stone LM, Finger TE. Mosaic analysis of the embryonic origin of taste buds. Chem Senses 1994;19:725–35.

Strek P, Litwin JA, Nowogrodzka-Zagorska M, Miodonski AJ. Microvasculature of the dorsal mucosa of human fetal tongue: a SEM study of corrosion casts. Anat Anz 1995;177:361–6.

Witt M, Kasper M. Immunohistochemical distribution of CD44 and some of its isoforms during human taste bud development. Histochem Cell Biol 1998;110:95–103.

Witt M, Kasper M. Distribution of cytokeratin filaments and vimentin in developing human taste buds. Anat Embryol 1999;199:291–9.

Witt M, Reutter K. Embryonic and early fetal development of human taste buds: a transmission electron microscopical study. Anat Rec 1996;246:507–23.

Witt M, Reutter K. Innervation of developing human taste buds. An immunohistochemical study. Histochem Cell Biol 1998;109:281–91.

16 SALIVARY GLANDS

DEVELOPMENT OF THE SALIVARY GLANDS

The three major pairs of salivary glands—parotid, submandibular, and sublingual—originate uniformly from oral epithelial buds invading the underlying mesenchyme (Fig. 16–1). All parenchymal (secretory) tissue of the glands arises from the proliferation of oral epithelium, which is either ectodermal (for the major glands) or endodermal (for the lingual glands) in origin. The stroma (capsule and septa) of the glands originates from mesenchyme that may be of either mesodermal or neural crest origin.

In all the salivary glands, after the initial formation of the buds, the epithelial cell cord elongates to form the main duct primordium, which invades the subepithelial stroma. At the distal end of this solid mass is a terminal bulb; this is the anlage of the intralobular salivary parenchyma. Branching produces arborization, and each branch terminates in one or two solid end bulbs. Elongation of the end bulbs follows, and lumina appear in their centers, transforming the end bulbs into terminal tubules. These tubules join the canalizing ducts (which are forming in the epithelial cord) to the peripheral acini. Canalization results from the mitosis of the outer layers of the cord being faster than that of the inner cell layers, and canalization is completed prior to lumen formation beginning in the terminal bulbs. Necrosis or apoptosis of cord cells as a mechanism of canalization has never been observed. Canalization is complete by the 6th month post conception.

The lining epithelium of the ducts, tubules, and acini differentiates both morphologically and functionally. Contractile myoepithelial cells arise from neural crest ectomesenchyme to surround the acini. Myoepithelial cells dif-

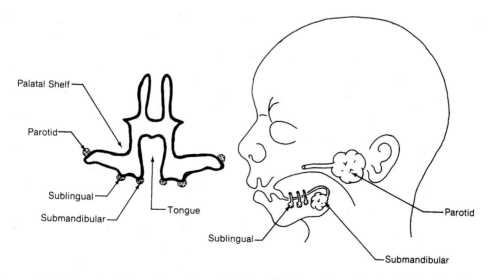

Figure 16–1 Schemata of the major salivary glands budding from the oral cavity. Their origins from the mouth are retained through their excretory ducts. The coronal sectional view through the mouth is shown on the left.

ferentiate at the time of onset of fetal secretory activity in the acini and achieve their full complement coincident with completion of the adult acinar-intercalated duct pattern at 24 weeks post conception in the submandibular gland and 35 weeks in the parotid gland. Interaction between epithelia, mesenchyme, nerves, and blood vessels is necessary for complete functional salivary gland morphogenesis. Autonomic innervation of the parenchymal cells is a key event in salivary gland development. Sympathetic-nerve stimulation is necessary for acinar differentiation whereas parasympathetic-nerve stimulation is important for overall gland growth.

The parotid gland buds are the first to appear, at the 6th week after conception. They appear on the inner cheek near the angles of the mouth and then grow back towards the ear. The maxillary and mandibular prominences merge, displacing the opening of the duct on the inside of the cheek to some distance dorsally from the corner of the mouth. In the "par-otid" or ear region, the epithelial cord of cells branches between the divisions of the facial nerve and canalizes to provide the acini and ducts of the gland. The ductal and acinar system is embedded in a mesenchymal stroma that is organized into lobules, and the whole gland becomes encapsulated by fibrous connective tissue. The parotid gland duct, repositioned upward, traces the path of the embryonic epithelial cord in the adult. The parotid ducts are canalized at 10 weeks post conception, the terminal buds are canalized at 16 weeks, and secretions commence at 18 weeks.

The submandibular salivary gland buds appear late in the 6th week as a grouped series, forming epithelial outgrowths on either side of the midline in the linguogingival groove of the floor of the mouth at the sites of the future papillae. An epithelial cord proliferates dorsally into the mesenchyme beneath the developing mylohyoid muscle, turning ventrally while branching and canalizing, to form the acini and duct of the submandibular gland. Differentiation of the acini starts at 12 weeks; serous secretory activity starts at 16 weeks, increases until the 28th week, and then diminishes. The serous secretions during the 16th to 28th weeks contribute to the amniotic fluid and contain amylase and possibly nerve and epidermal growth factors. Growth of the submandibular gland continues postnatally with the formation of mucous acini. The mesenchymal stroma separates off the parenchymal lobules and provides the capsule of the gland.

The sublingual glands arise in the 8th week post conception as a series of about 10 epithelial buds just lateral to the submandibular gland anlagen. These branch and canalize to provide a number of ducts that open independently beneath the tongue.

A great number of smaller salivary glands arise from the oral ectodermal and endodermal epithelium and remain as discrete acini and ducts scattered throughout the mouth. Labial salivary glands (on the inner aspect of the lips) arise during the 9th week post conception and are morphologically mature by the 25th week.

Failure of bud canalization to form ducts before acinar salivary secretion commences results in retention cysts.

Agenesis of the large salivary glands is rare.

THE JUXTAORAL ORGAN OF CHIEVITZ

This isolated organ of Chievitz appears in the adult as a tiny (7 to 17 mm long) white solid strand resembling a nerve, lying ventrodorsally in the cheek between the buccotemporal fascia and the parotid duct penetration of the buccinator muscle. It arises in the embryo as an oral epithelial invasion at the corners of the mouth, developing earlier than the anglagen of the parotid gland. It is closely associated with the buccal branch of the mandibular nerve that innervates it, but it loses its connection with the buccal sulcus and becomes embedded in a dense connective-tissue sheath. Although it may be a sensory receptor, its function is unknown.

Selected Bibliography

Adi MM, Chisholm DM, Waterhouse JP. Histochemical study of lectin binding in the human fetal minor salivary glands. J Oral Pathol Med 1995;24:130–5.

Chi JG. Prenatal development of human major salivary glands. Histological and immunohistochemical characteristics with reference to adult and neoplastic salivary glands. J Korean Med Sci 1996;11:203–16.

Chisholm DM, Adi MM. A histological, lectin and S-100 histochemical study of the developing prenatal human sublingual salivary gland. Arch Oral Biol 1995;40:1073–6.

D'Andrea V, Malinovsky L, Biancari F, et al. The Chievitz juxtaparotid organ. G Chir 1999;20:213–7.

Denny PC, Ball WD, Redman RS. Salivary glands: a paradigm for diversity of gland development. Crit Rev Oral Biol Med 1997;8:51–75.

Espin-Ferra J, Merida-Velasco JA, Garcia-Garcia JD, et al. Relationships between the parotid gland and the facial nerve during human development. J Dent Res 1991;70:1035–40.

Garrett JR, Ekström J, Anderson LC, editors. Neural mechanisms of salivary gland secretion. Basel: Karger; 1999.

Guizetti B, Radlanski RJ. Development of the parotid gland and its closer neighboring structures in human embryos and fetuses of 19-67 mm CRL. Anat Anz 1996;178:503–8.

Guizetti B, Radlanski RJ. Development of the submandibular gland and its closer neighboring structures in human embryos and fetuses of 19-67 mm CRL. Anat Anz 1996;178:509–15.

Hayashi Y, Kurashima C, Takemura T, Hirokawa K. Ontogenic development of the secretory immune system in human fetal salivary glands. Pathol Immunopathol Res 1989;8:314–20.

Jaskoll T, Melnick M. Submandibular gland morphogenesis: stage-specific expression of TGF-8/EGF, IGF, TGFβ, TNF, and II-6 signal transduction in normal embryonic mice and the phenotypic effects of TGF-β2, TGF-β3 and EGF-R null mutations. Anat Rec 1999;256:252–68.

Lee SK, Hwang JO, Chi JG, et al. Prenatal development of myoepithelial cell of human submandibular gland observed by immunohistochemistry of smooth muscle actin and rhodamine-phalloidin fluorescence. Pathol Res Pract 1993;189:332–41.

Melnick M, Jaskoll T. Mouse submandibular gland morphogenesis: a paradigm for embryonic signal processing. Crit Rev Oral Biol Med 2000;11:199–215.

Merida-Velasco JA, Sanchez-Montesinos I, Espin-Ferra J, et al. Development of the human submandibular salivary gland. J Dent Res 1993;72:1227–32.

Müller M, Jasmin JR, Monteil RA, Loubiere R. Embryology and secretory activity of labial salivary glands. J Biol Buccale 1991;19:39–43.

Thrane PS, Rognum TO, Brandtzaeg P. Ontogenesis of the secretory immune system and innate defence factors in human parotid glands. Clin Exp Immunol 1991; 86:342–8.

Zenken W. Juxtaoral organ (Chievitz's organ). Morphology and clinical aspects. Munich: Urban and Schwartzenburg; 1982.

17 MUSCLE DEVELOPMENT

Myogenesis is first manifested by the expression of myogenic regulatory factors (MRFs) (including MyoD1, MYF5, MRF-4/herculin/Myf-6, MyHCs, and myogenin) that differentiate myofibers with contractile properties from the paraxial mesoderm. Myogenic populations arise from unsegmented head mesoderm and segmented (somitic) mesoderm. The unsegmented muscle progenitors have a prolonged and necessary interaction with neural crest cells for development and provide the extraocular and pharyngeal-arch muscles. The segmented mesoderm develops the neck, tongue, laryngeal, and diaphragmatic muscles.

Craniofacial voluntary muscles develop from paraxial mesoderm that condenses rostrally as incompletely segmented somitomeres and segmented somites of the occipital and rostral cervical regions (Fig. 17–1). The myomeres of the somitomeres and the myotomes of the somites form primitive muscle cells termed *myoblasts*; these divide and fuse to form multinucleated myotubes that cease further mitosis and thus become myocytes (muscle fibers). Most muscle fibers develop before birth but increase in number and size in early infancy. Motor nerves establish contact with the myocytes, stimulating their activity and further growth by hypertrophy; failure of nerve contact or activity results in muscle atrophy.

Myogenic cells are spatially patterned by their intimately surrounding connective tissues. Muscles in the craniocervical regions derive their investing

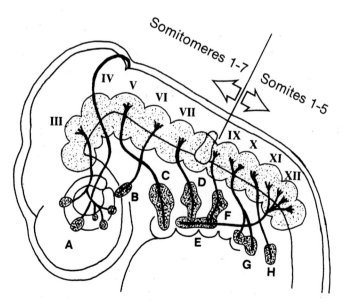

Figure 17–1 Origins of craniofacial muscles and their nerve supplies. Nerves: III, oculomotor; IV, trochlear; V, mandibular trigeminal; VI, abducens; VII, facial; IX, glossopharyngeal; X, vagus; XI, spinal accessory; XII, hypoglossal. Muscle groups: A, ocular; B, lateral rectus (ocular); C, masticatory; D, facial; E, glossal; F, pharyngeal; G, laryngeal; H, nuchal.

connective-tissue components from three sources. Neural crest tissue provides the epimysium, perimysium, and endomysium surrounding the myocytes of the extrinsic ocular, glossal, and all pharyngeal-arch skeletal muscles; the connective tissues of the laryngeal muscles arising from the first and second (occipital) somites are derived from postotic lateral plate mesoderm; and the connective-tissue components of the axial cervical muscles (trapezius and sternomastoid) are of somitic origin.

TABLE 17–1 Craniofacial Muscle Origins and Innervations

Mesodermal Origin	Muscles	Innervation (Cranial Nerve)
Somitomeres 1,2	Superior, inferior, and medial ocular recti; inferior oblique of eye	Oculomotor (III)
Somitomere 3	Superior oblique of eye	Trochlear (IV)
Somitomere 4	1st-arch masticatory muscles	Trigeminal (V)
Somitomere 5	Lateral ocular rectus	Abducens (VI)
Somitomere 6	2nd-arch facial muscles	Facial (VII)
Somitomere 7	3rd-arch stylopharyngeus	Glossopharyngeal (IX)
Somites 1,2	Laryngeal muscles	Vagus (X)
Somites 1–4	Tongue muscles	Hypoglossal (XII)
Somites 3–7	Sternomastoid, trapezius	Accessory (XI)

The craniofacial muscles are derived from the seven somitomeres and the seven most-rostral somites, gaining their cranial innervation sequentially (Table 17–1). Four extrinsic ocular muscles (superior, medial, inferior rectus, and inferior oblique) derive from the first two somitomeres, supplied by the oculomotor (third cranial) nerve. The superior oblique ocular muscle arises from the third somitomere, innervated by the trochlear (fourth cranial) nerve. The fourth somitomere myomere invades the first pharyngeal arch to provide the four muscles of mastication (masseter, temporalis, and medial and lateral pterygoids), innervated by the trigeminal (fifth cranial) nerve. The lateral rectus ocular muscle derives from the fifth somitomere, supplied by the abducent (sixth cranial) nerve. The sixth somitomere myomere invades the second pharyngeal arch to provide the facial muscles supplied by the facial (seventh cranial) nerve. The seventh somitomere forms the third pharyngeal-arch muscle, the stylopharyngeus, innervated by the glossopharyngeal (ninth cranial) nerve.

The myotomes of the first four (occipital) somites invade the fourth, fifth, and sixth pharyngeal arches, carrying their vagal (tenth cranial) and spinal accessory (eleventh cranial) nerves to provide the extrinsic and intrinsic laryngeal muscles. The hypoglossal cord, derived from the occipital somites (1 to 4) and supplied by the hypoglossal (twelfth cranial) nerve, migrates into the tongue region to form the intrinsic and extrinsic glossal muscles and contributes to the laryngeal muscles. Myotomic derivatives of the third to seventh somites, innervated by the spinal accessory nerve, form the sternomastoid and trapezius muscles.

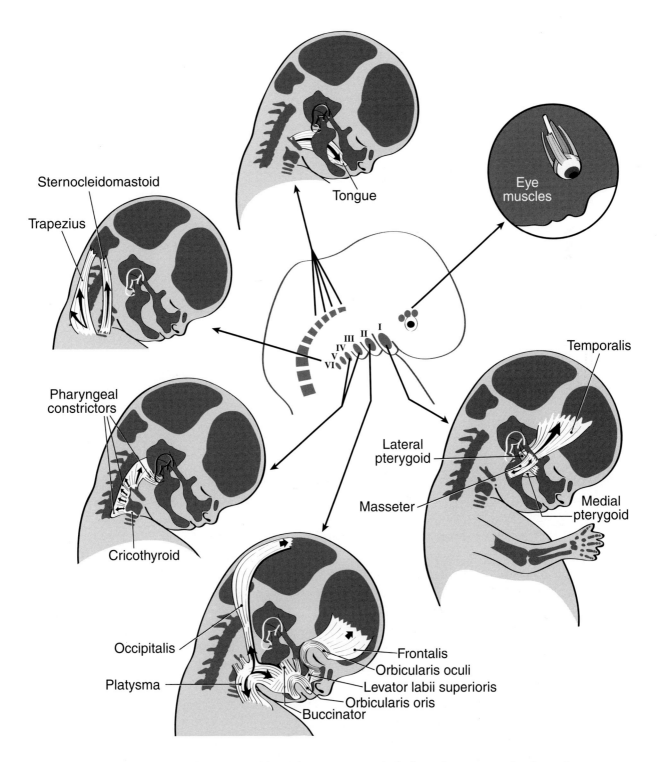

Figure 17–2 Schematic description of the embryonic origins of (clockwise from upper right) the ocular, masticatory, facial, pharyngeal, neck, and tongue muscles from somitomere, pharyngeal, and somite sources.

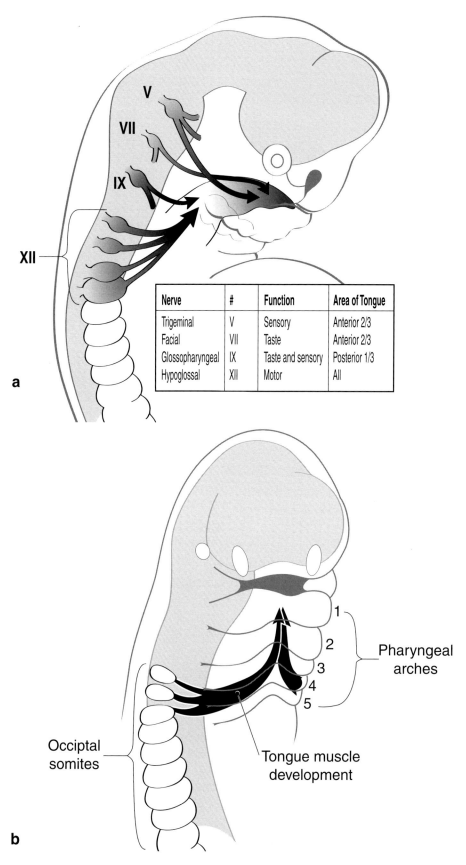

Nerve	#	Function	Area of Tongue
Trigeminal	V	Sensory	Anterior 2/3
Facial	VII	Taste	Anterior 2/3
Glossopharyngeal	IX	Taste and sensory	Posterior 1/3
Hypoglossal	XII	Motor	All

Figure 17–3 (*a*) Schematic depiction of the origin of the tongue muscles from the occipital somite myotomes. (*b*) The path of their migration is traced by the path of the hypoglossal nerve (XII).

The mesenchyme of the pharyngeal arches gives rise to special visceral (striated) musculature, innervated by special visceromotor cranial-nerve fibers that are under voluntary control. The transition from the specially striated visceral muscles of the mouth and pharynx to the "normal" unstriated (smooth) visceral muscle of the gut takes place in the esophagus, where voluntary control of food ingestion is lost.

The mesenchyme of the first pharyngeal arch, which phylogenetically is associated with the jaws, gives rise primarily to the muscles of mastication and some swallowing muscles. The second-arch mesenchyme provides the muscles of facial expression,* and the mesenchyme of the third, fourth, and fifth or sixth arches merges into the palatofaucial, pharyngeal, and laryngeal muscle groups (see p. 57 for details). The tongue, pharyngeal, and laryngeal muscles are of somitic origin and arise from ocipital somites 1 to 5 (Figs. 17–2 and 17–3; also see Fig. 17–1 in Chapter 17 and Fig. 15–2 in Chapter 15).

The orofacial muscles are the first to develop in the body, in keeping with the cephalocaudal sequence of fetal development. The genioglossus and geniohyoid muscles are the first premuscle masses to differentiate from occipital and cervical myotomic mesenchyme, at 32 to 36 days of age. The facial premuscle masses are formed between the ages of 8 and 9 weeks, menstrual age. (Menstrual age is 2 weeks more than the true age [ie, fertilization age] of the fetus. All subsequent ages mentioned in this chapter, unless designated post conception, are menstrual ages.) After migration, all the facial muscles are in their final positions by 14½ weeks. The mylohyoid muscle and the anterior belly of the digastric, which form the floor of the mouth, are the earliest of the muscles of the first pharyngeal arch to differentiate. The mylohyoid muscle initially attaches to the ventral border of Meckel's cartilage but later migrates dorsally to attach to the fetal mandible.

Of the palatal muscles, the tensor veli palatini is the first to develop from the first pharyngeal arch, as a mesenchymal condensation within the vertical palatal shelves at 40 days post conception. Next, the levator veli palatini and palatopharyngeus, derived from the fourth pharyngeal arch, develop simultaneously at 45 days. The uvular muscle develops at the time the palatal shelves fuse, by mesenchymal migration from the fourth pharyngeal arch. The palatoglossus muscle, also derived from the fourth pharyngeal arch, is the last palatal muscle to differentiate.

Second-arch mesenchyme destined to form the facial musculature is not initially subdivided into distinct muscle masses. Migration of the differentiating premyoblasts and early myoblasts extends from the region of the second pharyngeal arch in sheetlike laminae. The superficial lamina spreads from a location caudal to the external acoustic meatus in all directions and also around the meatus into the temporal, occipital, cervical, and mandibular regions. Migration of the second-arch myoblasts into the mesenchyme of the merged maxillary and mandibular prominences provides the important suck-

*The hyoid arch muscles, phylogenetically associated with the gill (pharyngeal) arches that regress in mammalian development, are adapted to the new mammalian function of facial expression. Fish and reptiles have no muscles of facial expression.

ling buccal and labial muscles. Differentiation of the premuscle masses, the development of boundaries, and the gaining of attachments now take place to distinguish the delicate superficial mimetic muscles of the face. The deep mesenchymal lamina condenses to become the stapedius muscle, the posterior belly of the digastric muscle, and the stylohyoid muscle.

The masticatory muscles differentiate as individual entities from first-arch mesenchyme, migrate, and gain attachment to their respective sites of origin on the cranium and sites of insertion on the mandible. The masseter and medial pterygoid have little distance to migrate, but their growth and attachments are closely associated with the mandibular ramus, which undergoes remodeling throughout the early, active growth period. As a consequence, these muscles must continually re-adjust their insertions and (to a much lesser extent) their sites of origin. The insertion of the lateral pterygoid into the head and neck of the rapidly remodeling mandibular condyle requires its constant reattachment, together with elongation concomitant with spheno-occipital synchondrosal growth, which synchondrosis intervenes between the origin and insertion of the muscle. The temporalis muscle's attachment to the temporal fossa stretches a considerable distance from its site of mandibular coronoid insertion as the muscle becomes employed in mastication. Its insertion also has to reattach constantly to the rapidly resorbing anterior border of the ramus and coronoid process during the most active growth period. The attachments of the buccinator muscle to the maxilla and mandible also require re-adjustment as the alveolar processes grow.

The histogenesis and morphogenesis of muscles and nerves influence each other; as the muscle masses form, the nerve and blood supplies to them differentiate. Nerve and vascular connections, established at the time of muscle-fiber development, persist even after the muscles have migrated from their sites of origin. This explains the long and sometimes tortuous paths that nerves and arteries may follow in the adult body; the wide paths of distribution of the facial nerve and the facial artery to the mimetic facial muscles are examples. Functional muscular activities begin as soon as neurologic reflex paths are established.

Muscle fibers gain their attachments to bone some time after their differentiation. The migration of muscles and ligaments relative to their bony attachments is a consequence of periosteal growth. The attachment of muscles to bones has some influence on bone formation, particularly as the muscles become functional and exert forces that invoke Wolff's law of bone response. Hypertrophy of muscles is associated with enlargement of correlated skeletal units; muscle atrophy commonly induces a like response in the associated bones.

The earliest muscle movement is believed to be reflex in origin, not spontaneous. Muscular response to a stimulus first develops in the perioral region, as a result of tactile cutaneous stimuli applied to the lips, indicating that the trigeminal nerve is the first cranial nerve to become active; the earliest movements in response to such exteroceptive stimuli have been elicited at 7½ weeks of menstrual age. (Myelinization, an indicator of nerve activity, appears first in the trigeminal nerve at 12 weeks but is not complete until the age of 1 to 2 years.) Spontaneous muscle movements are believed to begin only at 9½ weeks of menstrual age. Stroking the face of the 7½-week-old embryo produces a reflex bending of the head and upper trunk away from the stimulus, as a total neuromuscular response. This early contralateral avoidance reaction recapitulates the phylogenetically protective reflexes of primitive creatures, replaced later by a positive ipsilateral response to a stimulus.

Stimulation of the lips of the fetus at 8½ weeks results in incomplete but active reflex opening of the mouth in conjunction with all of the neuromuscular mechanisms sufficiently mature to react at this age. From 8½ to 9½ weeks of age, mouth opening forms part of a total contralateral reflex response to a stimulus, with lateral head and trunk flexion and movement of the rump and all four extremities. Mouth opening without concomitant head or extremity movements can be elicited only much later, at about 15½ weeks. Mouth closure is initially passive, but it is active and rapid after the 11th week as a result of the initiation of muscle stretch reflex activity. Swallowing begins at 12½ weeks in association with extension reflexes. At 13 to 14 weeks, early activity of the facial muscles may be manifested by a sneering expression in response to eyelid stimulation: the angle of the mouth is retracted, the lateral part of the upper lip is elevated, and the nasal ala on the ipsilateral side is raised (not bilaterally, as occurs postnatally). These early motor capabilities are unrelated to emotions. The spread of facial muscle activity is portrayed by the ability of the fetus to squint and scowl at 15 weeks. Tongue movements may begin as early as 12½ weeks, active lip movements begin at 14½ weeks, and the gag reflex can be elicited at 18½ weeks.

The early differentiation of the mylohyoid and digastric muscles would account for the early mouth-opening ability and may be essential to normal development. The withdrawal of the tongue from between the vertical palatal shelves (see p. 115) and the development of synovial cavities in the temporomandibular joint (see p. 141) may depend on these early mouth movements.

From 10 weeks post conception onward, mouth-opening reflexes become progressively less associated with a total lateral body reflex response to a stimulus, indicating the development of inhibitory-nerve pathways. However, head movements remain strongly associated with mouth movements even into the postnatal period, accounting for the "rooting reflex" whereby perioral stimulation leads to ipsilateral head rotation, which is associated with suckling in the infant. Another remnant of the total reflex response is the grasp reflex when an infant suckles.

Complex suckling movements involving mouth opening, lip protrusion, and tongue movements are not manifested spontaneously until 24 weeks of menstrual age although individual components of the movement can be elicited by stimulation about the mouth much earlier. Intrauterine thumb sucking has been demonstrated as early as 18 weeks. Crying may start between the 21st and 29th weeks post conception, reflecting the related muscle activities of the larynx and spasmodic inhalation and exhalation by the thoracic-cage musculature. Full swallowing and suckling that permit survival occur at only 32 to 36 weeks of fetal age. Some preliminary earlier swallowing occurs as early as 12

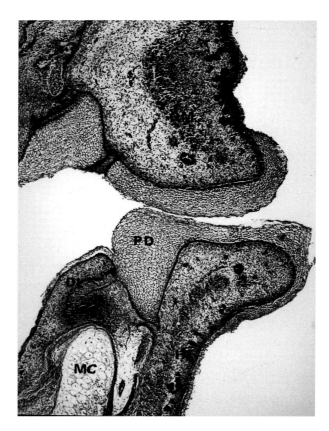

Figure 17–4 Paramedian sagittal section of the lips of a 12-week-old fetus. Note the nature of the multilayered periderm (PD), the developing orbicularis oris muscle (OM), the dental lamina (DL), and Meckel's cartilage (MC). Hair follicles (HF) are forming in the cutaneous areas. (× 56 original magnification) (Courtesy of Dr. R. R. Miethke)

weeks, when the fetus literally drinks the amniotic fluid in which it is bathed.* The coordinated effective combination of suckling and swallowing is an indicator of neurologic maturation that is particularly important for the survival of the premature infant. Respiratory movements may be elicited by a stimulus as early as 13 weeks, but the spontaneous rhythmic respiration necessary for survival does not occur until much later. Increasingly complex muscle movements producing mastication and speech depend upon the development of the appropriate reflex proprioceptive mechanisms.

The cutaneous covering of the lips of the fetus is sharply delineated from the adjacent skin and oral mucosa (Fig. 17–4). The primitive epithelium of the vermilion surface of the lip forms a distinctive multilayered periderm that is shed in utero. At birth, the surface of the infant's lips is subdivided into a central highly mobile suckling area characterized by fine villi (pars villosa), distinct from an outer smooth zone (pars glabra), and an inner vestibular zone (pars

---

*The importance of this early swallowing is indicated by the excess amniotic fluid (hydramnios) found in the amniotic sacs of fetuses unable to swallow because of esophageal atresia. Near term, the normal fetus will swallow as much as 200 to 600 mL of amniotic fluid per day. The swallowed amniotic fluid is absorbed by the gut, from whence it is carried by the fetal bloodstream to the placenta. It is then passed on to the maternal body for elimination. Interestingly, amniotic fluid is not normally inspired into the lungs of the fetus.

mucosa) (Fig. 17–5). The villous portion of the infant lip is adhesive, more so than the glabrous or vestibular portions; during suckling, this adhesion may result from swelling of the blood vessels in the villi, establishing an airtight seal around the nipple.

The conspicuous philtrum of the neonatal upper lip gradually loses its clarity during childhood, the central depression becoming shallower in the adult. The rare phenomenon of double lip (either upper or lower) results from hypertrophy of the inner pars villosa and an exaggerated boundary line demarcating it from the outer pars glabra. Congenital fistulae of the lower lip—usually bilateral, seldom unilateral, and occasionally median—are rare. Their occurrence may be genetically determined as an autosomal dominant trait in Van der Woude syndrome, located on chromosome 1q32-q41.

With use, muscles increase in size due to hypertrophy of their individual fibers; conversely, muscle disuse results in atrophy. At birth, the suckling muscles of the lips (orbicularis oris) and cheeks (buccinators) are relatively better developed than the muscles of mastication (Fig. 17–6). Indeed, at birth, mobility of the face is limited to the eyelids, the middle of the lips, and the slight corrugation in the areas of the forehead and mental protuberance. Between birth and adulthood, the facial muscles increase fourfold in weight, and the muscles of mastication increase sevenfold in weight. The masseter and medial pterygoid are better developed at birth than the temporalis and lateral pterygoid muscles. The buccinator muscle is prominent in the cheek of the neonate;

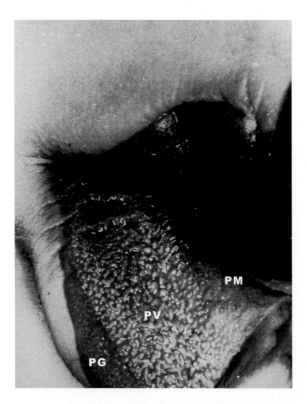

Figure 17–5 Lips and commissure of the mouth of a 39-week-old fetus. In the lower lip, note the outermost smooth pars glabra (PG) that narrows towards the commissure. The central pars villosa (PV) is covered with fine villi. The inner vestibular zone, the pars mucosa (PM), is continuous with the vestibule of the mouth. (Approximately x4 original magnification). (Courtesy of Dr. R. R. Miethke)

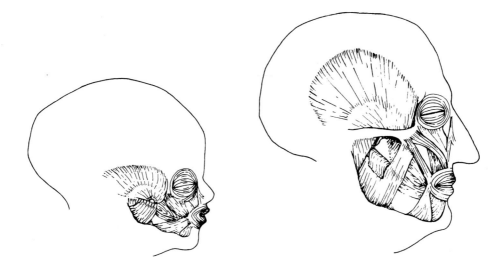

Figure 17–6 Muscle development at birth and in adulthood. In infancy, the suckling facial muscles are relatively better developed than the muscles of mastication. In adulthood, the muscles of mastication are more strongly developed than the facial muscles. Compare the area of attachment of the temporalis muscle in the infant and the adult.

its powerful suckling capabilities are enhanced by a large subcutaneous adipose mass, forming a "sucking pad" that prevents collapse of the cheeks during suckling.* The tongue musculature is well developed at birth, and the tongue has a wide range of movement.

All of the complex interrelated orofacial movements of suckling, swallowing, breathing, and gagging are reflex in origin rather than learned and constitute unconditioned congenital reflexes necessary for survival. Conditioned acquired reflexes develop with the maturation of the neuromuscular apparatus and are generally learned as habits. The development of abnormal patterns of movement ("bad" habits) is likely the result of conditioned fetal reflex activity developing out of sequence or the omission of a specific response to a sequential triggering stimulus.

Until the primary first molars erupt, the infant swallows with jaws separated and tongue thrust forward, predominantly using the facial muscles (orbicularis oris and buccinators) innervated by the facial nerve. This pattern, known as the infantile swallow, is an unconditioned congenital reflex. Contrary to the action in adults, the infant's lips suck during swallowing and make stronger movements than the tongue. After the eruption of the posterior primary teeth at 18 months of age onward, the child tends to swallow with the teeth brought together by masticatory muscle action, without a tongue thrust. This mature swallow is an acquired conditioned reflex and is intermingled with the infantile swallow during a transition period. As the child grows older, variation in the pattern decreases as the adult swallowing pattern is increasingly adopted. The movements of the mature swallow are primarily of those muscles innervated

*The buccal fat pad of Bichat is peculiarly loose in texture and is bounded by a connective-tissue capsule. The fat in the pad persists even in emaciation, indicating its structural and mechanical function rather than fat storage.

by the trigeminal nerve (ie, the muscles of mastication and the mylohyoid). Once the facial-nerve musculature has been relieved of its swallowing duties, it is better able to perform the delicate mimetic activities of facial expression and speech that are acquired from 18 months onward.

The infant's cry is a nonconditioned reflex, which accounts for its lack of individual character and sporadic nature. Speech, on the other hand, is a conditioned reflex, which differs among individuals but is regular by virtue of the sophisticated control required.

Mastication is a conditioned reflex, learned by initially irregular and poorly coordinated chewing movements. (The proprioceptive neuromuscular spindles are much sparser in the lateral pterygoid muscle than in the other masticatory muscles, accounting for its uncoordinated behavior.) The proprioceptive responses of the temporomandibular joint and the periodontal ligaments of the erupting dentition establish a stabilized chewing pattern aligned to the individual's dental intercuspation.

The conversion of the infantile swallow into the mature swallow, of infantile suckling into mastication, and of infantile crying into speech are all examples of the substitution of conditioned reflexes acquired with maturation for the unconditioned congenital reflexes of the neonate. Superimposed upon these reflex movements are voluntary activities under conscious control, acquired by learning and experience.

The maturation of normal neuromuscular reflexes and the development of a proper equilibrium of muscular forces during orofacial growth is necessary for normal jaw morphology and dental occlusion. Tongue movements and lip and cheek pressures guide erupting teeth into normal occlusion. The retention of the teeth-apart tongue-thrusting infantile pattern of swallowing into childhood creates abnormal myofunctional pressures upon the teeth, resulting in a characteristic "open-bite" pattern of malocclusion. Muscle malfunctioning, either by their hyper- or hypotonicity, and particularly of the orbicularis oris-buccinator-tongue complex, results in dental malocclusion. The pressures exerted by these muscles partly determine the form of the dental arches.

Selected Bibliography

Burdi AR, Spyropoulous MN. Prenatal growth patterns of the human mandible and masseter muscle complex. Am J Orthod 1978;74:380.

Ferrario VF, Sforza C, Schmitz JH, et al. Normal growth and development of the lips: a 3-dimensional study from 6 years to adulthood using a geometric model. J Anat 2000;196:415–23.

Gasser RF. Development of the facial muscles in man. Am J Anat 1967;120:357.

Humphrey T. The development of the mouth opening and related reflexes involving the oral area of human fetuses. Ala J Med Sci 1968;5:126–57.

Humphrey T. The relation between human fetal mouth opening reflexes and closure of the palate. Am J Anat 1969;125:317–44.

Humphrey T. Development of oral and facial motor mechanisms in human fetuses and their relation to craniofacial growth. J Dent Res 1971;50:1428.

Miethke RR. Zur Anatomie der Ober- und Unterlippe zwischen dem 4 intrauterinen Monat und der Geburt. Gegenbaurs Morphol Jahrb 1977;123:424.

Mooney MP, Siegel MI, Kimes KR, et al. Development of the orbicularis oris muscle in normal and cleft lip and palate human fetuses using three-dimensional computer reconstruction. Plast Reconstr Surg 1988;81:336.

Noden DM, Marcucio R, Borycki A-G, Emerson CP Jr. Differentiation of avian craniofacial muscles: I. Patterns of early regulatory gene expression and myosin heavy chain synthesis. Dev Dyn 1999;216:96–112.

Radlanski RJ, Renz H, Tabatabi A. Prenatal development of the muscles in the floor of the mouth in human embryos of 6.9–76 mm CRL. Ann Anat 2000;182:98.

Rodriguez-Vazquez JF, Merida-Velasco JR, Arraez-Aybar LA, Jimenez-Collado J. Anatomic relationships of the orbital muscle of Muller in human fetuses; Radiol Surg Anat 1998;20:341–4.

Rodriguez-Vazquez JF, Merida-Velasco JR, Jimenez-Collado J. Orbital muscle of Müller: observations on human fetuses measuring 35-150 mm. Acta Anat 1990;139:300–3.

Trainor PA, Tam PP. Cranial paraxial mesoderm and neural crest cells of the mouse embryo: co-distribution in the craniofacial mesenchyme but distinct segregation in the branchial arches. Development 1995;121:2569–82.

Zahng L, Yoshimura Y, Hatta T, Otani H. Myogenic determination and differentiation of the mouse palatal muscle in relation to the developing mandibular nerve. J Dent Res 1999;78:1417–25.

18 SPECIAL-SENSE ORGANS

The organs of the special senses of olfaction, gustation, vision, balance, and hearing are all located in the craniofacial complex. Parts of these special-sense organs initially arise in a similar manner. (The organs of the special sense of gustation, the taste buds [see p. 162], differ from the other special-sense organs in this respect.) Underlying cranial neural crest tissue induces localized areas of surface ectoderm to thicken and differentiate into distinct placodes. The subsequent fates of the olfactory, lens, and otic placodes will be briefly described individually. (The development of the external apparatus of the nose, however, has been considered together with the development of the face [see p. 39].)

THE NOSE

The specialized olfactory epithelium of the nose appears as the olfactory (nasal) placodes (see Fig. 3–5 in Chapter 3) on the inferolateral aspects of the frontonasal prominence, toward the end of the somite period. The "sinking" of the olfactory placodes into the depths of the olfactory pits causes the specialized olfactory epithelium of each placode to be located ultimately in the lateral walls of the upper fifth of each nasal cavity. The olfactory nerve cells connect with the olfactory bulb of the brain through the cribriform plate of the ethmoid bone.

THE EYE

The eye is derived from surface ectoderm, neural ectoderm, neural crest tissue, and mesoderm. The light-sensitive portion of the eye, the retina, is a direct outgrowth from the forebrain, projecting bilaterally as the optic vesicles, which are connected to the brain by the optic stalks (Fig. 18–1). The neuroectodermal optic vesicles induce their overlying surface ectoderm to thicken. This forms the lens placodes, each of which invaginates in its center by the development of peripheral folds, which fuse to convert it into a closed *lens vesicle*. These vesicles sink beneath the surface ectoderm; initially hollow, they become filled with lens fibers to form the lenses. The optic vesicles, also, invaginate partly to form the double-layered optic cups, and the optic stalks become the optic nerves. The outer layer of the optic cup acquires neural crest pigmentation to become the pigmented layer of the retina, and the inner layer differentiates into the light-sensitive nervous layer (Fig. 18–2).

Meningeal ectomesenchyme (of neural crest origin) surrounding the optic cups and lenses forms the sclera and choroid over the cups, the ciliary bodies at the margins of the cups, and the cornea over the lenses. Mesoderm invades the optic cups to form the vitreous body and the transient hyaloid artery. The extrinsic muscles of the eye are derived from the prechordal somitomeres (see p. 172).

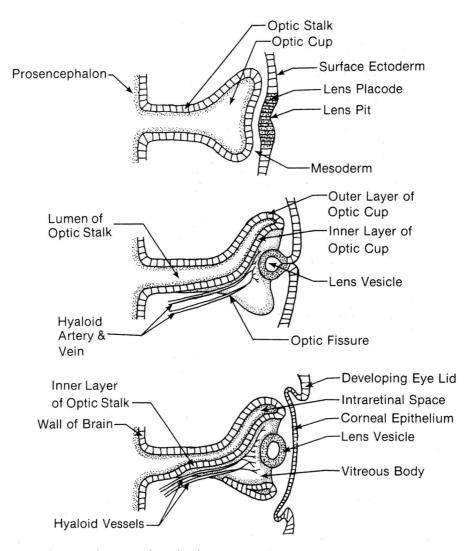

Figure 18–1 Schematic depiction of eye development at various stages.

The cutaneous ectoderm overlying the cornea forms the conjunctiva. Ectodermal folds develop above and below the cornea; with their central core of mesenchyme, they form the eyelids. The eyelids close at the end of the 8th week post conception and remain closed until the 7th month after conception.

The eyes migrate from their initially lateral positions toward the midline of the face, and over- and undermigration produce anomalies of facial appearance (hypotelorism and hypertelorism) (see p. 38). The visual ability of the neonate is exceedingly poor. The ability to resolve visual details is some 40 times less than that of adults, with uncoordinated movements of the eyes and no depth appreciation. Visual acuity improves to nearly adult level by the end of the 1st year.

THE EAR

The three parts of the ear—external, middle, and internal—arise from separate and diverse embryonic origins, reflecting the complicated phyloge-

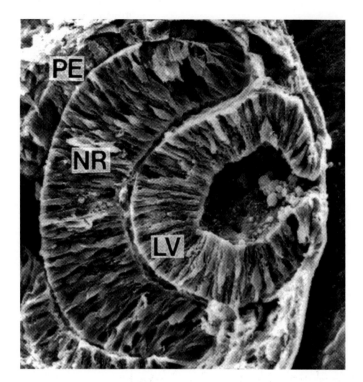

Figure 18–2 Scanning electron micrograph of a sectioned optic cup and lens vesicle of an 11-day-old mouse embryo, approximating a 36-day-old human embryo. The lens vesicle (LV) overlies the neural retina (NR) adjacent to the pigmented epithelium (PE). (Courtesy of Drs. K. K. Sulik and G. C. Schoenwolf)

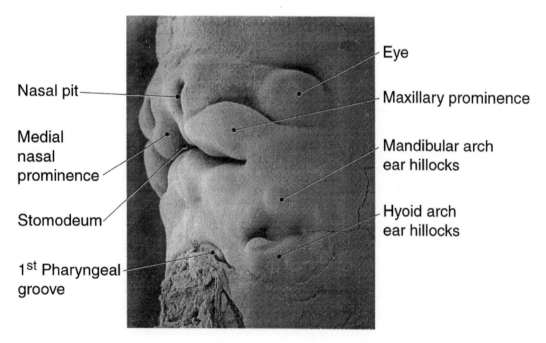

Figure 18–3 Scanning electron micrograph of a 6-week-old human embryo, showing auricle development from the first two pharyngeal arches. (Courtesy of Dr. K. K. Sulik)

netic history of the adaption of the primitive pharyngeal-arch apparatus for hearing and balance.

The external ear forms around the first pharyngeal groove (see Fig. 5–1 in Chapter 5), which deepens to become the external acoustic meatus, initially located in the mandibulocervical region. The auricle develops as a series of six

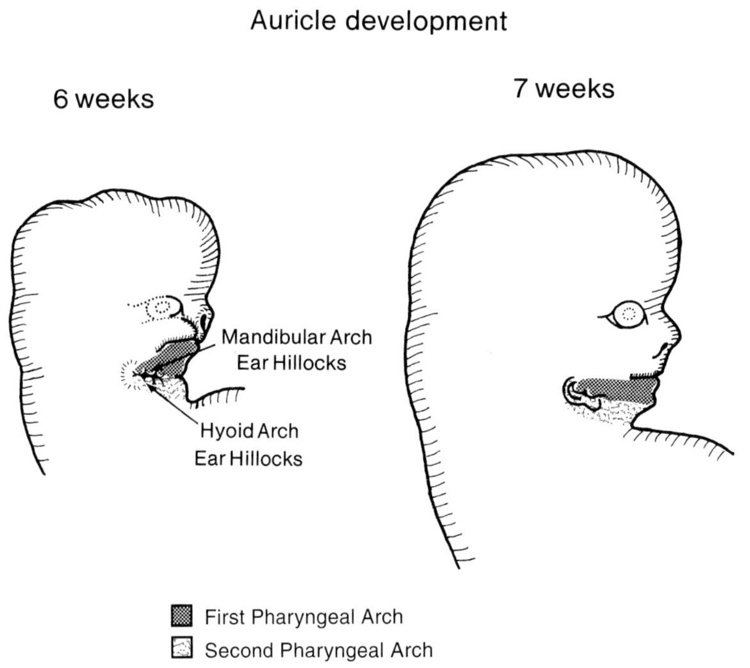

Auricle development

6 weeks   7 weeks

Mandibular Arch
Ear Hillocks

Hyoid Arch
Ear Hillocks

▨ First Pharyngeal Arch
▧ Second Pharyngeal Arch

Figure 18–4 Auricle development from the first two pharyngeal arches.

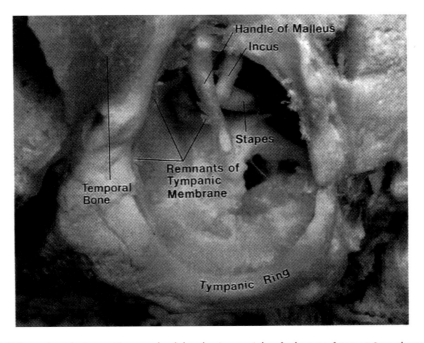

Figure 18–5 Scanning electron micrograph of developing auricle of a human fetus at 9 weeks post conception. (Courtesy of Dr. K. K. Sulik)

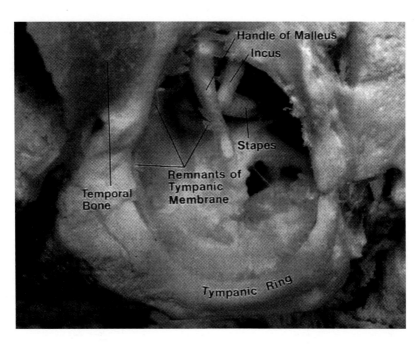

Figure 18–6 Photograph of the tympanum in a neonatal skull. The tympanic membrane has been torn away to reveal the three ear ossicles in situ. The base of the stapes is in the fenestra vestibuli, and the fenestra cochleae is seen below it. Note the superficial location of the middle ear in the skull of the newborn, due to the absence of a bony external acoustic meatus. (× 3 original magnification)

swellings or hillocks surrounding the dorsal aspect of the first pharyngeal groove. Three of the hillocks develop from the first (mandibular) pharyngeal arch, and the other three develop from the second (hyoid) pharyngeal arch (Figs. 18–3 and 18–4). Differential growth and fusion of the hillocks by the end of the 8th week produces the characteristic shape of the auricle (Fig. 18–5). The auricle and external acoustic meatus appear to migrate cranially from their original cervical location to reach their "normal" position by the 4th month post conception, largely due to mandibular growth. Elastic cartilage differentiates in the mesenchyme around the external acoustic meatus.

The tympanic ring of the temporal bone forms the boundaries of the tympanic membrane, which closes off the external acoustic meatus from the middle ear (Fig. 18–6). At birth, the external acoustic meatus is shallow; therefore, the tympanic ring and tympanic membrane are located superficially. Also, both the ring and the membrane are markedly oblique in the neonate; these structures achieve nearly adult size by birth and thus require this orientation for their accommodation within the still fetal-sized acoustic meatus from the late fetal stage onward. Outward growth of the bony tympanic ring and cartilage of the meatus deepens the meatus during infancy and childhood and allows the adult orientation of the tympanic membrane and (consequently) the ossicular chain.

The middle ear develops from the tubotympanic recess derived from the first pharyngeal pouch (see p. 63). The endodermal lining of the tympanic recess comes into proximity with the ectodermal lining of the external acoustic meatus and, with a thin layer of intermediate mesoderm, forms the tympanic membrane. Expansion of the tympanic cavity surrounds and envelops the

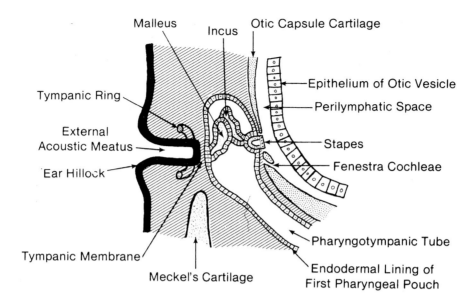

Figure 18–7 Schematic illustration of early stage (5 weeks post conception) of ear development. The external ear (auricle and external acoustic meatus) forms around the first pharyngeal groove. The middle ear develops from the first pharyngeal pouch, and the ear ossicles develop from the first (malleus and incus) and second (stapes) pharyngeal arches. The internal ear develops from the otic vesicle.

chain of three ear ossicles developing from the first and second pharyngeal-arch cartilages (Fig. 18–7) (see Chapter 4). The ossicles thus appear to lie within the tympanic cavity although they actually lie outside it, surrounded by the pharyngeal endodermal membrane. The tympanic cavity achieves nearly adult size by 37 weeks post conception. Further expansion of the tympanic cavity postnatally gives rise to the mastoid air cells.

The muscles attaching to the auditory tube (the tensor veli palatini and the tensor tympani) differentiate respectively at 12 and 14 weeks post conception. These muscles (with the later-developing salpingopharyngeus) function at birth to open the tube. Fluid clearance is difficult in the neonate due to the narrow cylindrical lumen and the horizontal orientation of the tube. By contrast, the adult tube is angled downward medially, with a funnel-shaped lumen facilitating middle-ear drainage. Swallowing aids the establishment of hearing, which normally is impaired for the first 2 days after birth.

The malleus and incus are derived from the dorsal end of the cartilage of the first pharyngeal arch (see p. 54), the joint between them representing the primitive jaw joint (see Chapter 13). (The incus arises from the separated end of Meckel's cartilage that corresponds with the pterygoquadrate cartilage of infra-mammalian vertebrates.) The stapes derives partly from the dorsal end of the second-arch cartilage, in which three ossification centers appear. Ossification of the ear ossicles begins in the 4th month post conception and proceeds rapidly to form functional bones by the 25th week post conception.* These are the first

---

*Ossification of these bones is endochondral, but the anterior process of the malleus forms independently in membrane bone. After birth, this anterior mallear process shrinks to less than one-third of its prenatal length. Initial ossification appears at 17 weeks post conception on the long process of the incus, followed by the neck of the malleus and spreading to the manubrium and head. Stapedial ossification begins at its base at the 18th week.

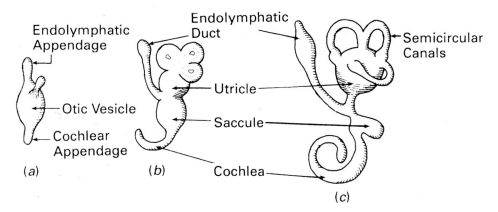

Figure 18–8 Stages of internal ear development from the otic vesicle at (*a*) 5 weeks, (*b*) 6 weeks, and (*c*) 7 weeks post conception.

bones in the body to attain their ultimate size. The cartilage of the otic capsule breaks down around the footplate of the stapes to form the oval window. Failure of this chondrolysis is a source of one form of congenital deafness.

The tensor tympani muscle, attaching to the malleus, is derived from the first pharyngeal arch and is innervated by the mandibular division of the trigeminal nerve of that arch. The stapedius muscle, attached to the stapes, is derived from the second pharyngeal arch and is accordingly innervated by the facial nerve of that arch.

The internal ear arises from the otic placode at 21 to 24 days post conception. This is the first sensory organ to begin development; this development is initiated by neural crest induction of surface ectoderm. Epithelioecto-mesenchymal interactions between the otic placode and subjacent mesenchyme are necessary for the histogenesis and morphogenesis of the labyrinth of the inner ear. Invagination of the placode creates the otic cup, and apposition of its folded margins forms the otic vesicle or otocyst that sinks beneath the surface ectoderm. Subsequent complicated configurations of the otocyst give rise to the endolymphatic duct and sac, the saccule and utricle, the three semicircular canals, and the cochlear duct. Together, these form the membranous labyrinth (Fig. 18–8). The otocyst induces chondrogenesis in the surrounding mesenchyme, to form the otic capsule. The surrounding cartilage of the otic capsule conforms to the intricate shape of the membranous labyrinth and forms the bony labyrinth when intramembranous ossification of the modiolus occurs. The rigidity imparted by the location of the labyrinths, deeply embedded within bone, determines the fixed orientation of the three semicircular canals on each side to each other and also to the head, allowing the development of balance and centrifugal senses. The capacity of the cochlea to respond to vibratory stimuli is established between 24 and 25 weeks post conception.

ANOMALIES OF DEVELOPMENT

Anomalies of the ear include anotia and microtia, afflicting the auricle (which is absent or reduced) and resulting in nonpatency of the external acoustic meatus (atresia). The auditory tube is hypoplastic in nearly all cases of cleft palate.

A more severe facial anomaly is synotia, in which the ears are abnormally located ventrally in the upper part of the neck (see Fig. 3–21 in Chapter 3) and which is almost invariably accompanied by agnathia (see p. 47). This association has been attributed to the absence of the neural crest tissue that normally migrates into the lower anterior part of the face. Not only does the mandible fail to form, but the otocysts that form the ear occupy a cervical position that is normally separated by mandibular neural crest ectomesenchyme. The presence and growth of the mandible appears to be a factor in the location of the ears.

Selected Bibliography

Achiron R, Gottlieb Z, Yaron Y, et al. The development of the fetal eye: in utero ultrasonographic measurements of the vitreous and lens. Prenatal Diagn 1995;15:155–60.

Ars B. Organogenesis of the middle ear structures. J Laryngol Otolol 1989;103:16–21.

Bagger-Sjoback D. Embryology of the human endolymphatic duct and sac. ORL J Otorhinolaryngol Relat Spec 1991;53:61–7.

Barishak YR. Embryology of the eye and its adnexae. Dev Ophthalmol 1992;24:1–142.

Bremond-Gignac DS, Banali K, Deplus S, et al. In utero eyeball development study by magnetic resonance imaging. Surg Radiol Anat 1997;19:319–22.

Costa-Neves M, Rega R de M, Wanderley SS. Quantitative growth of the eye in the human fetus. Ital J Anat Embryol 1992;97:55–9.

Declau F. Development of the human external auditory canal. Acta Otorhinolaryngol Belg 1995;49:95–9.

Declau F, Moeneclaey L, Marquet J. Normal growth pattern of the middle ear cleft in the human fetus. J Laryngol Otolol 1989;103:461–5.

Denis D, Burguiere O, Burillon C. A biometric study of the eye, orbit, and face in 205 normal human fetuses. Invest Ophthalmol Vis Sci 1998;39:2232–8.

Denis D, Faure F, Volot F, et al. Ocular growth in the fetus. 2. Comparative study of the growth of the globe and the orbit and the parameters of fetal growth. Ophthalmologica 1993;207:125–32.

Denis D, Righini M, Scheiner C, et al. Ocular growth in the fetus. 1. Comparative study of axial length and biometric parameters in the fetus. Ophthalmologica 1993;207:117–24.

Fekete DM, Development of the vertebrate ear: insights from knockouts and mutants. Trends Neurosci 1999;22:263–9.

Ferrario VF, Sforza C, Ciusa V, et al. Morphometry of the normal human ear: a cross sectional study from adolescence to mid-adulthood. J Craniofac Genet Dev Biol 1999;19:226–33.

Fini ME, Strissel KJ, West-Mays JA. Perspectives on eye development. Dev Genet 1997;20:175–85.

Gasser RF, Shigihara S, Shimada K. Three-dimensional development of the facial nerve path through the ear region in human embryos. Ann Oto Rhino Laryngol 1994;103:395–403.

Gill P, Vanhook J, Fitzsimmons J, et al. Fetal ear measurements in the prenatal detection of trisomy 21. Prenat Diagn 1994;14:739–43.

Goldstein I, Tamir A, Zimmer EZ, Itskovitz-Eldor J. Growth of the fetal orbit and lens in normal pregnancies. Ultrasound Obstet Gynecol 1998;12:175–9.

Karmody CS, Annino DJ Jr. Embryology and anomalies of the external ear. Facial Plast Surg 1995;11:251–6.

Lambert PR, Dodson EE. Congenital malformations of the external auditory canal. Otolaryngol Clin North Am 1996;29:741–60.

Lang T, Arnold WH. 3-D reconstructions of the developmental stages of the membranous labyrinth in human embryos and fetuses. Ann Anat 2000;182:99.

Miodonski AJ, Gorczyca J, Nowogrodzka-Zagorska M, et al. Microvascular system of the human fetal inner ear: a scanning electron microscopic study of corrosion casts. Scanning Microsc 1993;7:585–94.

Morsli H, Tuorto F, Choo D, et al. Otx1 and Otx2 activities are required for the normal development of the mouse inner ear. Development 1999;126:2335–45.

Ng M, Linthicum FH. Morphology of the developing human endolymphatic sac. Laryngoscope 1998;108:190–4.

Nishikori T, Hatta T, Kawauchi H, Otani H. Apoptosis during inner ear development in human and mouse embryos: an analysis by computer-assisted three-dimensional reconstruction. Anat Embryol 1999;200:19–26.

Oguni M, Setogawa T, Matsui H, et al. Timing and sequence of the events in the development of extraocular muscles in staged human embryos: ultrastructural and histochemical study. Acta Anat 1992;143:195–8.

Oguni M, Setogawa T, Otani H, et al. Development of the lens in human embryos: a histochemical and ultrastructural study. Acta Anat 1994;149:31–8.

Peck JE. Development of hearing. Part II. Embryology. J Am Acad Audiol 1994;5:359–65.

Piza J, Northrop C, Eavey RD. Embryonic middle ear mesenchyme disappears by redistribution. Laryngoscope 1998;108:1378–81.

Pujol R, Lavigne-Rebillard M, Uziel A. Development of the human cochlea. Acta Otolaryngol Suppl 1991;482:7–12.

Salminen M, Meyer BI, Bober E, Gruss P. Neutrin 1 is required for semicircular canal formation in the mouse inner ear. Development 2000;127:13–22.

Shimizu T, Salvador L, Hughes-Benzie R, et al. The role of reduced ear size in the prenatal detection of chromosomal abnormalities. Prenat Diagn 1997;17:545–9.

Sohmer H, Freeman S. Functional development of auditory sensitivity in the fetus and neonate. J Basic Clin Physiol Pharmacol 1995;6:95–108.

Torres M, Giraldez F. The development of the vertebrate inner ear. Mech Dev 1998;71:5–21.

Ulatowska-Blaszyk K, Bruska M. The cochlear ganglion in human embryos of developmental stages 18 to 19. Folia Morphol (Warsz) 1999;58:29–35.

Vazquez E, San Jose I, Naves J, et al. P75 and Trk oncoproteins expression is developmentally regulated in the inner ear of human embryos. Int J Dev Biol 1996;1:77S–8S.

19 DEVELOPMENT OF THE DENTITION

ODONTOGENESIS

Teeth developed in primitive fishes when placoid scales overlying their jaws were adapted to form dermal denticles. This phylogenetic dermal origin of teeth is reflected in the embryonic development of human teeth; although they develop while submerged beneath the oral gingival epithelium, human teeth partly originate from ectodermal tissue. Teeth are derived from ectoderm and mesoderm (two of the primary germ layers), with a neural crest contribution. The enamel of teeth is derived from oral ectoderm, and neural crest tissue provides material for the dentine, pulp, and cementum. The periodontium is of both neural crest and mesodermal origin.

Prior to any histologic evidence of tooth development, the alveolar nerves grow into the jaws; their branches form plexuses adjacent to sites of ectomesenchymal condensation, suggesting a possible neural inductive influence. Ectomesenchyme derived from the neural crest is the primary material of odontogenesis. A great number of genes associated with signaling molecules and epithelial-mesenchymal interactions are expressed in developing teeth.

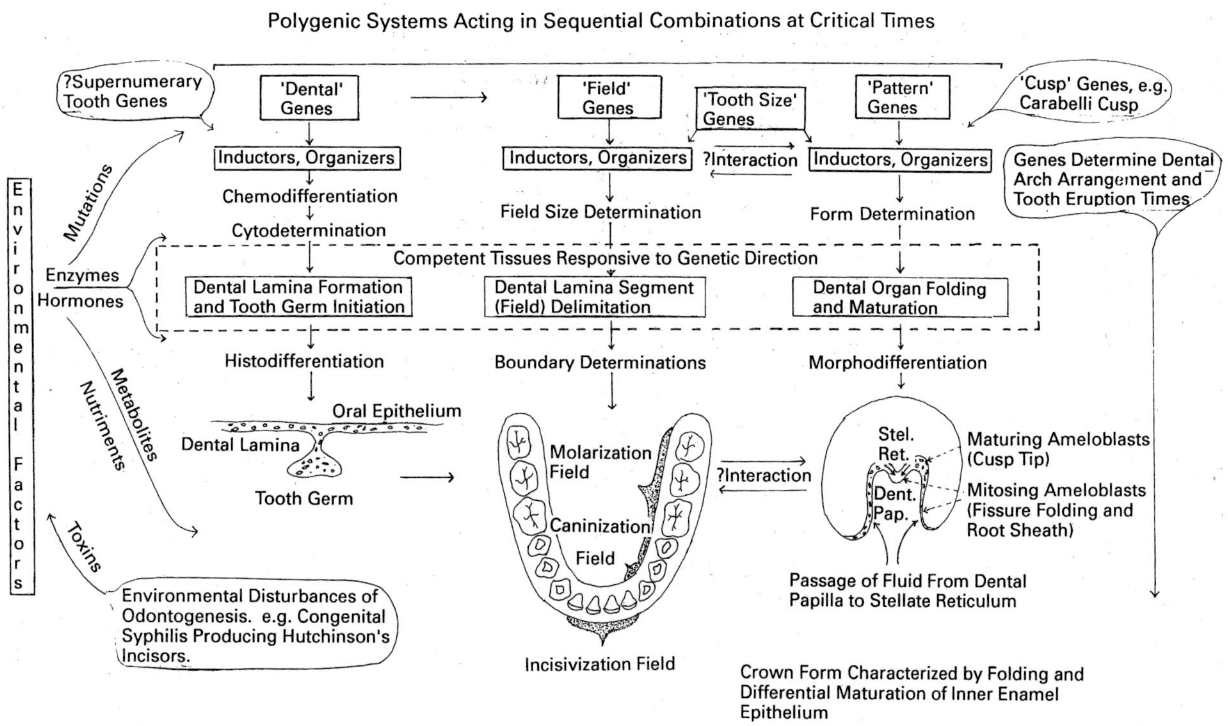

Figure 19–1 Postulated mechanism of odontogenesis. Stel. Ret., stellate reticulum; Dent. Pap., dental papilla. (Reproduced by permission of the Canadian Dental Association)

Signaling molecules from PAX9, MSX1, nerve growth factor (NGF), the sonic hedgehog (SHH) gene, fibroblast growth factor (FGF), bone morphogenetic protein (BMP), and distal-less (Dlx) and wingless (Wnt)* families regulate early stages of tooth morphogenesis. These gene products are organizers of odontogenesis, producing structures whose distinct dental patterns are formed by these genes.

Inductive interaction between neural crest tissue and pharyngeal endoderm (and subsequently with oral ectoderm) is followed by proliferation of the oral ectoderm. Fibroblast growth factors and their receptors are expressed in several successive key steps in tooth formation, regulated by reciprocal tissue interactions. These interactions produce the first morphologically identifiable manifestation of tooth development, the dental lamina. Later, the neural crest cells form the individual dental papillae, determining the ultimate number of teeth (Figs. 19–1 and 19–2).

Potential odontogenic tissue can be identified as early as the 28th day of development (fertilization age) as areas of ectodermal epithelial thickening on the margins of the stomodeum at the same time that the oropharyngeal membrane disintegrates. The oral epithelium thickens on the inferolateral borders of the maxillary prominences and on the superolateral borders of the mandibular arches where the two join to form the lateral margins of the stomodeum. Additional and initially separate odontogenic epithelium arises at the inferolateral borders of the frontonasal prominence on the 35th day of development, providing four sites of origin of odontogenic epithelium for the maxillary dentition. Thus, it seems that the anterior maxillary teeth derive from the frontonasal prominence and that the posterior maxillary teeth originate from the maxillary prominences. The mandibular dentition also develops four initial odontogenic sites in the mandibular arches, two on each side.

The four maxillary dental laminae coalesce on the 37th day, by which age the mandibular dental laminae have fused. The upper and lower dental laminae now form continuous horseshoe-shaped plates. Local proliferations of the

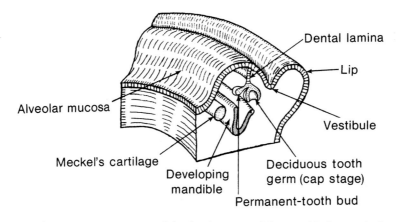

Figure 19–2 Schematic representation of the development of the mandibular vestibular and dental laminae.

*The terms "distal-less" and "wingless" refer to orthologous genes first described as mutations in *Drosophila* (fruit flies), hence their names.

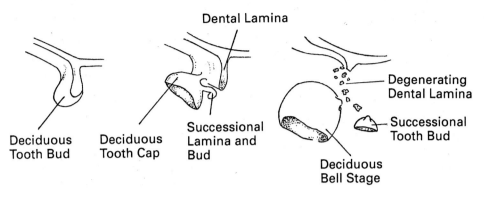

Figure 19–3 The bud (left), cap (middle), and bell (right) stages of tooth development.

dental laminae are induced (in a constant genetically determined sequence) into the subjacent mesenchyme at locations corresponding to the dental papillae that are forming from neural crest cells. Fibroblast growth factors act as mitogens for the odontogenic cells and stimulate the expression of MSX1, a transcription factor, needed for normal tooth development. The positioning of teeth depends upon the discrete locations of competent mesenchyme responding to a continuous inductively active epithelium. The discontinuous distribution of nerve endings along the dental lamina and their possible influence on migrating neural crest cells account for ectomesenchymal localization beneath the oral epithelium with which interaction occurs. The ectodermal projections form the primordia of the enamel organs, and (together with the

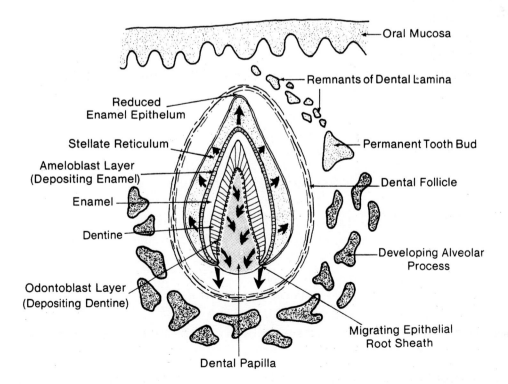

Figure 19–4 The developing deciduous teeth, showing directions of dental-tissue deposition and growth.

dental papillae) account for the subsequent submerged development of the teeth.

The vestibular lamina develops buccally and labially to the dental laminae. The vestibular laminae split the outer margins of the stomodeum into buccal segments that become the cheeks and lips and into lingual segments in which the teeth and alveolar bone develop. A sulcus (the vestibule of the mouth) develops between the buccal and lingual segments. Unsplit segments of the vestibular lamina remain as labial frenula (singular, frenulum).

Ten tooth germs (matching the number of deciduous teeth) develop in each jaw. Later, the tooth germs of the permanent succedaneous teeth appear lingually to each deciduous-tooth germ. The primordia of the permanent molar teeth develop from distal extensions of the dental laminae. Each tooth germ consists of an enamel organ and a dental papilla surrounded by a dental follicle or sac. The dental papilla (of neural crest origin) and dental follicle (of mesodermal origin) are respectively the anlagen of the dental pulp and part of the periodontal apparatus.

During its development, each enamel organ changes from its initial small bud shape, enlarging by rapid mitosis of the basal cells into a cap shape and later cupping into a large bell shape; the three stages of enamel organ development are designated by these shapes (Fig. 19–3). Concomitant with these morphologic alterations, histodifferentiation occurs within the enamel organ. The external layer forms the outer enamel epithelium, a layer of cuboidal cells subjacent to the developing follicle. The stellate reticulum, composed of stellate cells set in a fluid matrix, constitutes the central bulk of the early enamel organ. The indented inner layer, lining the dental papilla, forms the inner enamel epithelium, part of which differentiates into the transient secretory columnar ameloblasts that form enamel. Lining a portion of the stellate reticular surface of the inner enamel epithelium is a squamous cellular condensation, the stratum intermedium, that probably helps the ameloblasts form enamel. The inner and outer enamel epithelia form the cervical loop, elongating into Hertwig's epithelial root sheath, which outlines the root(s) of the tooth by enclosing more and more of the dental papilla (Figs. 19–4 and 19–5). The number of roots of a tooth is determined by the subdivision (or lack thereof) of the root sheath into one, two, or three compartments.

The inner enamel epithelium interacts with the ectomesenchymal cells of the dental papilla, whose peripheral cells differentiate into odontoblasts. The formation of dentine by the odontoblasts both precedes and is necessary for the induction of preameloblasts into ameloblasts to produce enamel (Fig. 19–6). The inner enamel epithelium of the root sheath induces odontoblast differentiation but, lacking a stratum intermedium, fails to differentiate itself into enamel-forming ameloblasts, accounting for the absence of enamel from the roots. Cementum forms on dentine adjacent to the sites of disintegration of the outer enamel epithelium of the root sheath. The fragmentation of the root sheath, due to programmed cell death (apoptosis), leaves clusters of cells—the epithelial rests of Malassez—in the periodontal ligament. These rests are the source of potential periodontal cysts. The fibers in the initial

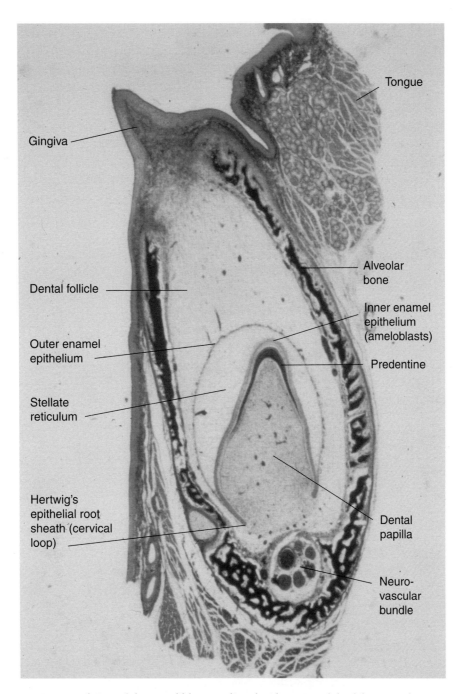

Figure 19–5 Sectioned view of the mandible, revealing deciduous-tooth bud, bone, and neurovascular bundle (× 25 original magnification). (Courtesy of Professor Dr. W. Arnold)

cementum derive solely from fibers of the pre-existing dental follicle that form the first principal fibers of the periodontal ligament.

The ameloblasts of the inner enamel epithelium and the adjacent odontoblasts together form a bilaminar membrane, which spreads by mitosis under genetic control and varies among the tooth germs in different areas. Different foldings of the bilaminar membrane are dictated by signaling molecules emanating from the enamel knot in the dental organ. Enamel knots are signaling centers regulating the epithelial folding that specifies the varied shapes of incisors, canines, premolars, and molars. The confined space of the dental follicle imposes folding upon the enlarging amelodentinal membrane. The ameloblasts secrete a protein matrix of amelogenins and enamelins that later mineralize as enamel rods or prisms as they retreat from the membrane. Concomitantly, the odontoblasts secrete the collagen matrix of predentine, which later calcifies into dentine (see Figs. 19–5 and 19–6). Dentine deposition is a continuous process throughout life. The dental papilla differentiates into the dental pulp, the peripheral cells into odontoblasts, and the remaining cells into fibroblasts. Enamel formation is restricted to the pre-eruptive phase of odontogenesis and ends with the deposition of an organic layer, the enamel cuticle. The enamel organ collapses after deposition of this cuticle. The inner and outer enamel epithelia together with the remains of the stratum intermedium form the reduced enamel epithelium, which later fuses with the overlying oral mucous membrane to initiate the pathway for eruption (Fig. 19–7).

Meanwhile, the mesenchyme surrounding the dental follicles becomes ossified, forming bony crypts in which the teeth develop and from which they are later to erupt. An investing mesenchymal layer of the dental follicle adja-

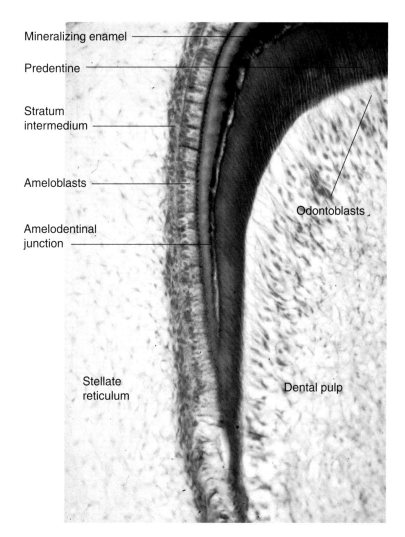

Mineralizing enamel

Predentine

Stratum intermedium

Ameloblasts

Amelodentinal junction

Odontoblasts

Stellate reticulum

Dental pulp

Figure 19–6 Histologic section of amelodentinal junction, depicting early predentine formation in a tooth bud. (× 125 original magnification) (Courtesy of Professor Dr. W. Arnold)

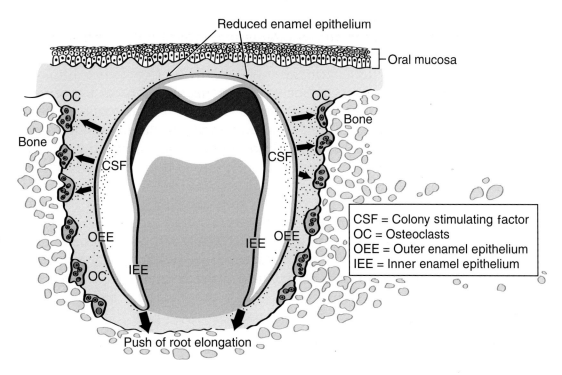

Figure 19–7 Schematic synopsis of various factors that may operate during tooth eruption.

cent to the cementum differentiates into the inner layer of the periodontal ligament by the development of collagen fibers. These fibers are already organized into inner, outer, and intermediate layers between cementum and bone. The periodontal ligament is the tissue through which orthodontic tooth movement is effected. Reorganization of the attachment apparatus (comprising cementum, periodontal fibers, and alveolar bone) is requisite to successful tooth movement during orthodontic treatment.

The anterior deciduous (incisor, canine, and first molar) tooth germs develop first, at the 6th week post conception; the second deciduous molar germs begin to appear at the 7th week. The anterior permanent (incisor, canine, and premolar) tooth germs bud from the lingual side of the corresponding deciduous enamel organs whereas the second deciduous and permanent molar tooth germs develop directly from backward extension of the dental lamina. The germs of the first permanent molars begin to develop at about the 16th week post conception; those of the second and third permanent molars do not appear until after birth. Formation of most of the permanent teeth is not complete until several years after birth; root formation for the third molars is not complete until about 21 years of age. In this respect, teeth have the most prolonged chronology of development of any set of organs in the body.

ERUPTION OF THE TEETH

The mechanisms by which teeth erupt have not been fully elucidated, and several processes have been proposed to explain the movement of teeth from their crypts into the oral cavity. The elongation of the root of a tooth during its development, and the growth of the pulp within it while the apical foramen is wide open, are likely to be sources of at least part of the eruptive force. The deposition of cementum upon the surface of the root would provide some slight eruptive movement once root formation was completed. The path of eruption ahead of the crown of a tooth would be guided by the remnants of the attachments of the dental follicle to the oral epithelium from which it originated (gubernacular cords). Blood pressure in the tissue around the root of a tooth and changes in the vascularity of the periodontal tissues have been implicated as eruptive forces.

Also, a form of functional-matrix activity stemming from interplay between the periodontal ligament and the hard tissues has been postulated. The proliferating connective tissue of the periodontal ligament or an accumulation of periodontal-tissue fluids resulting from increased vascular permeability would tend to separate tooth and bone and thereby provide an eruptive force. This is analogous to the pathologic state in which an inflamed edematous periodontal ligament pushes a tooth out of its socket although this may not be strictly comparable to physiologic eruption.

Another theory suggests that contraction of the obliquely orientated collagen fibers of the periodontal ligament produces a "pulling" force contrasting with most of the "pushing" forces indicated above. The traction of the periodontal ligament has been attributed to the contraction of fibroblasts; the presumed contraction of the fibroblasts of periodontal connective tissues has been likened to the contraction of scar tissue during wound healing. Contractile capabilities have been attributed to the fibroblasts (myofibroblasts) of the periodontal and cicatricial connective tissues.

An intact dental follicle is essential for eruption to occur. Cellular activity of the reduced enamel epithelium and the follicle initiates a cascade of signaling, by expressing epidermal and transforming growth factors. These cytokines stimulate the follicle cells to express colony-stimulating factors (CSFs), recruiting monocytes that fuse to form osteoclasts that (together with the proteases from the reduced enamel epithelium) resorb overlying alveolar bone, producing an eruption pathway for the tooth (see Fig. 19–7).

Tooth eruption results from a combination of several factors operating concomitantly, sequentially, or sporadically. The absence of any of the factors may be compensated for by another factor. Tooth eruption appears to be an intermittent rather than a continuous process, composed of alternating stages of movement and equilibrium. (Teeth that grow continuously—such as the incisors of rodents—erupt continuously throughout life.) Individual posteruptive tooth movement, producing migration and hypereruption, is subject to local factors of mastication or tooth disuse. The net eruptive force (eruption minus resistance) of a tooth is quite small, of the order of 5 g of pressure.

The eruption of the molar teeth is combined with their mesial drift, which ensures their contact with the anterior teeth and their interproximal contact with one another when erupted. This tendency to mesial drift during eruption would account also for the mesial impaction of unerupted teeth, in which forward movement is greater than eruptive (upward or downward) movement. Vertical tooth eruption not only contributes to the great increase in height of the face during childhood but also compensates for loss of facial height resulting from attritional wear of the occlusal surfaces of teeth. Protrusion of the anterior teeth may contribute to a dentally prognathic facial profile.

The regular sequence of tooth eruption suggests that it is under genetic control that programs the life cycle of the dental epithelium and follicle. Tooth eruption is highly subject to nutritional, hormonal, and disease states, and there is considerable intersubject variation in the age at which it occurs. Disturbances of the "normal" sequence and ages of tooth eruption contribute to the development of dental malocclusion and are consequently of significance to orthodontists.

At birth, the jaws contain the partly calcified crown of the 20 deciduous teeth, and the first permanent molars begin to calcify (Table 19–1). Eruption of the deciduous dentition, beginning at 7½ months of age on average, terminates at about 29 months. Dental eruption is then quiescent for nearly 4 years. At the age of 6 years, the jaws contain more teeth than at any other time: 48 teeth crammed between the orbits and the nasal cavity and filling the body of the mandible (Fig. 19–8). Between 6 and 8 years of age, all eight deciduous incisors are lost, and 12 permanent teeth erupt. After this extreme activity, there is a 2½-year quiet period, until 10½ years of age. Then, during the next 18 months, the remaining 12 deciduous teeth are lost, and 16 permanent teeth erupt.

The 6-year period of the mixed dentition from 6 to 12 years of age is the most complicated period of dental development and the one in which malocclusion is most likely to develop. A long and variable period (3 to 7 years) of quiescence follows before eruption of the four third molars completes the dentition. The third molars do not begin calcifying until the 9th year of age, and

TABLE 19–1 Chronology of Development and Eruption of Teeth

Tooth	Tooth Germ Completed	Calcification Commences	Crown Completed	Eruption Commences	Root Completed
Deciduous					
Incisors	12–16 wk pc	3–4 mo pc	2–4 mo	6–8 mo	1½–2 yr
Canines	12–16 wk pc	5 mo pc	9 mo	16–20 mo	2½–3 yr
1st molars	12–16 wk pc	5 mo pc	6 mo	12–15 mo	2–2½ yr
2nd molars	12–16 wk pc	6–7 mo pc	11–12 mo	20–30 mo	3 yr
Permanent					
Central incisors	30 wk pc	3–4 mo	4–5 yr	Max: 7–9 yr Mand: 6–8 yr	9–10 yr
Lateral incisors	32 wk pc	Max: 10–12 mo Mand: 3–4 mo	4–5 yr	7–9 yrs	10–11 yr
Canines	30 wk pc	4–5 mo	6–7 yr	Max: 11–12 yr Mand: 9–10 yr	12–15 yr
1st premolars	30 wk pc	1½–2 yr	5–6 yr	10–12 yr	12–14 yr
2nd premolars	31 wk pc	2–2½ yr	6–7 yr	10–12 yr	12–14 yr
1st molars	24 wk pc	Birth	3–5 yr	6–7 yr	9–10 yr
2nd molars	6 mo	2½–3 yr	7–8 yr	12–13 yr	14–16 yr
3rd molars	6 yr	7–10 yr	12–16 yr	17–21 yr	18–25 yr

Note: All dates are postnatal, except those designated post conception (pc).
Mand = mandible; Max = maxilla; wk = weeks; mo = months; yr = years.

their eruption from the 16th year onward heralds the completion of dentofacial growth and development.

All 12 permanent molars originate from identical sites in all four quadrants of the jaw. The upper molars develop within the maxillary tuberosity, three on each side, and the lower three molars of each side develop within the ascending ramus of the mandible. The first and second molars migrate forward from their sites of origin into the alveolar bone of the maxilla or mandible, from which they erupt to meet their antagonists.

Bone resorption of the anterior border of the mandibular ramus and bone deposition on the maxillary tuberosity create space for the eruption of the permanent molar teeth. Failure of adequate continued bone growth of the jaws during this eruption period for either genetic or environmental reasons precludes space for the full eruption of all the permanent teeth, resulting in mal-eruption, partly impacted eruption, or non-eruption of the last-formed teeth.

All the teeth in the jaws are carried downward, forward, and laterally as the face expands, except for the central incisors, which maintain their proximity to the median plane. The faster rate of tooth eruption is superimposed upon this slower bone movement, a combination of movements that determine dental and gnathoskeletal growth patterns. The continual tendency of the teeth to erupt and migrate means that this mechanism is constantly compensating for the attritional wear of teeth, to stabilize the vertical dimension of the face. Dental occlusion is maintained by a combination of bone remodeling and tooth eruption that reflects the neuromuscular actions of the orofacial apparatus.

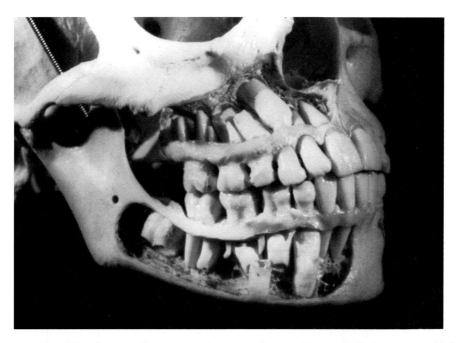

Figure 19–8 Mixed deciduous and permanent dentitions dissected in the skull of an 8-year-old child. Note the location of the unerupted permanent teeth in the bodies of the maxilla and mandible.

ANOMALIES OF DEVELOPMENT

Congenital absence of teeth (anodontia) may be total or (more frequently) partial, following a hereditary pattern involving individual teeth, or being part of a syndrome (eg, ectodermal dysplasia). Anodontia of varying severity afflicts some 20 percent of the population. A mutation of the PAX9 gene located on chromosome 14 (with an extra nucleotide in the gene) produces a smaller-than-normal PAX9 protein, leading to congenital absence of molars. Some types of teeth (eg, third molars) are frequently congenitally absent whereas others (eg, first molars and canines) are rarely so. Anomalous forms of teeth are extremely varied.

Defects of enamel (amelogenesis imperfecta) and dentine (dentinogenesis imperfecta) may be expressions of genetic autosomal dominant disorders or sporadic environmentally determined hypoplasia or hypomineralization of the hard tissues. Teeth are particularly sensitive to deficiencies of certain vitamins and hormones, to metabolic disturbances, to bacterial and viral infections, and to certain drugs (eg, fluorides and tetracyclines) during their formation. These agents inflict permanently retained lesions upon the forming hard tissues, providing a record of the timing of the occurrence.

Selected Bibliography

Dental enamel. Proceedings of a symposium. Ciba Found Symp (London) 1997;205:1–284. Chicester (NY): Wiley; 1997.

The third Carolina conference on tooth enamel formation. Chapel Hill, North Carolina. Adv Dent Res 1996;10:89–275.

Butler WT. Dentin matrix proteins and dentinogenesis. Connect Tissue Res 1995; 33:59–65.

Casasco A, Casasco M, Calligaro A, et al. Cell proliferation in developing human dental pulp. A combined flow cytometric and immunohistochemical study. Eur J Oral Sci 1997;105:609–13.

Chen Y, Bei M, Woo I, et al. Msx1 controls inductive signaling in mammalian tooth morphogenesis. Development 1996;122:3035–44.

Chiego DJ Jr. The early distribution and possible role of nerves during odontogenesis. Int J Dev Biol 1995;39:191–4.

Christensen LR, Mollgard K, Kjaer I, Janas MS. Immunocytochemical demonstration of nerve growth factor receptor (NGF-R) in developing human fetal teeth. Anat Embryol 1993;188:247–55.

Cobourne MT. The genetic control of early odontogenesis. Brit J Orthod 1999;26:21–8.

Cuisinier FJ, Steuer P, Senger B, et al. Human amelogenesis: high resolution electron microscopy of nanometer-sized particles. Cell Tissue Res 1993;273:175–82.

Fincham AG, Moradian-Oldak J, Simmer JP. The structural biology of the developing dental enamel matrix. J Struct Biol 1999;126:270–99.

Gibson CW. Regulation of amelogenin gene expression. Crit Rev Eukaryot Gene Expr 1999;9:45–57.

Gorczycz J, Litwin JA, Nowogrodzka-Zagorska M, et al. Microcirculation of human fetal tooth buds: a SEM study of corrosion casts. Eur J Morphol 1994;32:3–10.

Heikinheimo K. Stage-specific expression of decapentaplegic-Vg-related genes 2, 4, and 6 (bone morphogenetic proteins 2, 4, and 6) during human tooth morphogenesis. J Dent Res 1994;73:590–7.

Kettunen P. Fibroblast factors in tooth development. Dissertationes Biocentri Viikki Universitatis Helsingiensis. Helsinki: Yliopistopaino; 1999.

Kjaer I, Bagheri A. Prenatal development of the alveolar bone of human deciduous incisors and canines. J Dent Res 1999;78:667–72.

Kollar EJ. Odontogenesis: a retrospective. Eur J Oral Sci 1998;106 Suppl 1:2–6.

Lau EC, Slavkin HC, Snead ML. Analysis of human enamel genes: insights into genetic disorders of enamel. Cleft Palate J 1990;27:121–30.

Limeback H. Molecular mechanisms in dental hard tissue mineralization. Curr Opin Dent 1991;1:826–35.

Linde A, Goldberg M. Dentinogenesis. Crit Rev Oral Biol Med 1993;4:679–728.

Luukko K. Neuronal cells and neurotrophins in odontogenesis. Eur J Oral Sci 1998;1:80–93.

Maas R, Bei M. The genetic control of early tooth development. Crit Rev Oral Biol Med 1997;8:4–39.

Mark M, Lohnes D, Mendelsohn C, et al. Roles of retinoic acid receptors and of Hox genes in the patterning of the teeth and of the jaw skeleton. Int J Dev Biol 1995;39:111–21.

Marks SC Jr, Schroeder HE. Tooth eruption: theories and facts. Anat Rec 1996;245:374–93.

Mornstad H, Staaf V, Welander U. Age estimation with the aid of tooth development: a new method based on objective measurements. Scand J Dent Res 1994;102:137–43.

Peters H, Neubuser A, Balling R. Pax genes and organogenesis: Pax 9 meets tooth development. Eur J Oral Sci 1998;1:38–43.

Radlanski RJ, van der Linden FP, Ohnesorge I. 4D-computerized visualisation of human craniofacial skeletal growth and of the development of the dentition. Anat Anz 1999;181:3–8.

Robinson C, Brooks SJ, Shore RC, Kirkham J. The developing enamel matrix: nature and function. Eur J Oral Sci 1998;106 Suppl 1:282–91.

Simmer JP, Fincham AG. Molecular mechanisms of dental enamel formation. Crit Rev Oral Biol Med 1995;6:84–108.

Slavkin HC. Molecular determinants of tooth development: a review. Crit Rev Oral Biol Med 1990;1:1–16.

Smith CE. Cellular and chemical events during enamel maturation. Crit Rev Oral Biol Med 1998;9:128–61.

Stockton DW, Das P, Goldenberg M, et al. Mutation of PAX9 is associated with oligodontia. Nat Genet 2000;24:18–9.

Ten Cate AR. The role of epithelium in the development, structure and function of the tisues of tooth support. Oral Dis 1996;2:55–62.

Ten Cate AR. The development of the periodontium—a largely ectomesenchymally derived unit. Periodontol 2000 1997;13:9–19.

Thesleff I. Tooth morphogenesis. Adv Dent Res 1995; 9(3 Suppl):12.

Thesleff I, Sharpe P. Signalling networks regulating dental development. Mech Dev 1997;67:111–23.

Thesleff I, Vainio S, Jalkanen M. Cell-matrix interactions in tooth development. Int J Dev Biol 1989;33:91–7.

Tucker AS, Sharpe PT. Molecular genetics of tooth morphogenesis and patterning: the right shape in the right place. J Dent Res 1999;78:826–34.

Ulm MR, Chalubinski K, Ulm C, et al. Sonographic depiction of fetal tooth germs. Prenat Diagn 1995;15:368–72.

Ulm MR, Kratochwil A, Ulm B, et al. Three-dimensional ultrasonographic imaging of fetal tooth buds for characterization of facial clefts. Early Hum Dev 1999;55:67–75.

Vastardis H. The genetics of human tooth agenesis: new discoveries for understanding dental anomalies. Am J Orthod Dentofac Orthoped 2000;117:650–6.

Weiss K, Stock D, Zhao Z, et al. Perspectives on genetic aspects of dental patterning. Eur J Oral Sci 1998;106 Suppl 1:55–63.

Weiss KM, Stock DW, Zhao Z. Dynamic interactions and the evolutionary genetics of dental patterning. Crit Rev Oral Biol Med 1998;9:369–98.

Zeichner-David M, Diekwisch T, Fincham A, et al. Control of ameloblast differentiation. Int J Dev Biol 1995;39:69–92.

APPENDIX
Primary Germ Layers

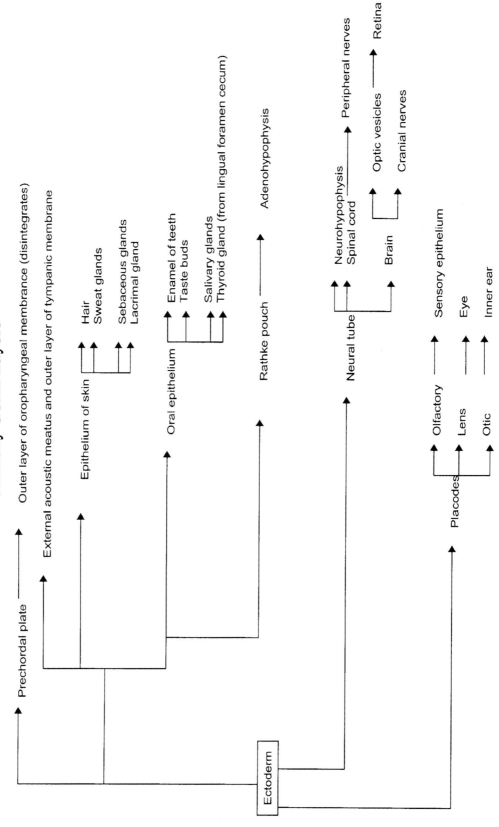

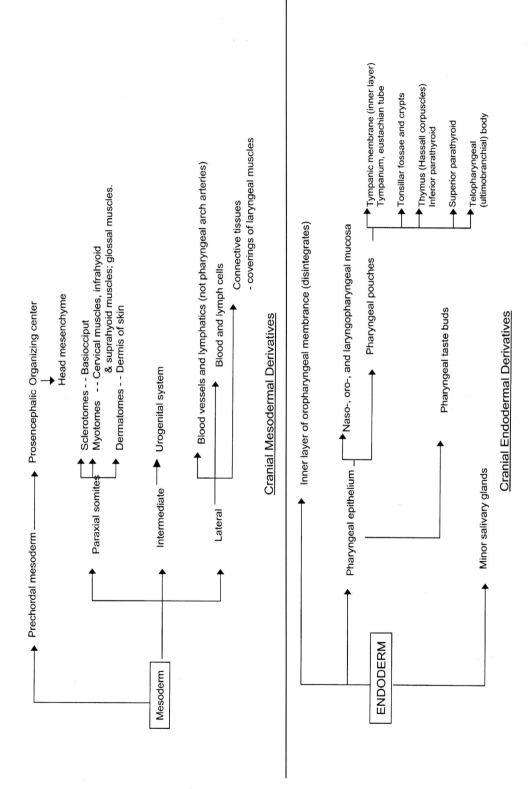

Cranial Mesodermal Derivatives

Cranial Endodermal Derivatives

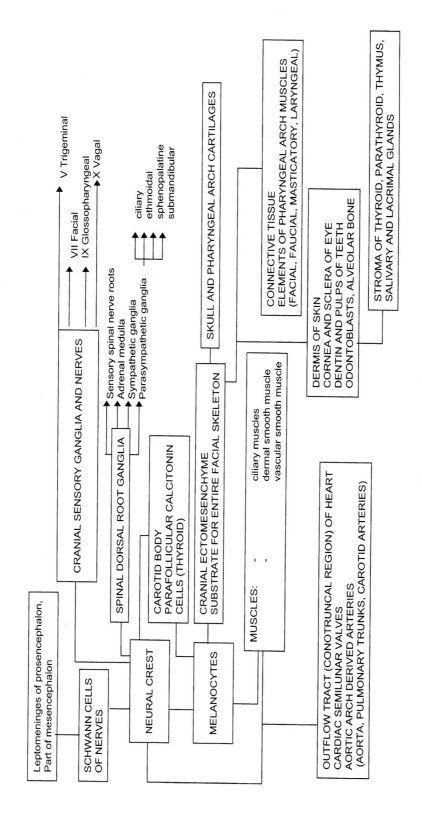

Neural Crest Derivatives

Derivatives of Germ Layers

From: G.H. Sperber "Craniofacial Abnormalities" in Potter's Pathology of the Fetus and Infant. E. Gilbert-Barness, Editor, C.V. Mosby Co., St. Louis, MO. With Permission.

GLOSSARY OF SELECTED TERMS

acalvaria	Absence of the calvaria.
acrania	Absence of the cranium.
adenohypophysis	Anterior lobe of the pituitary gland; derived from Rathke's pouch.
aglossia	Absence of the tongue.
agnathia	Absence of the mandible.
allantois	Fetal membrane, a diverticulum of the hindgut. Its blood vessels form the umbilical blood vessels.
ameloblast	Cell type giving rise to the enamel of teeth.
amelogenesis	Process of enamel production.
amnion	Fetal membrane enveloping the fetus.
anencephaly	Absence of the brain .
aneuploidy	Abnormal chromosome number; the basis of genetic defects.
ankyloglossia	Tongue-tie, an anomaly of tongue development.
ankylosis	An immobile or fixed joint.
anlage	Embryonic primordium of an organ.
anophthalmia	Absence of the eyes.
anotia	Absence of the external ears.
aortic arches	Arteries encircling the embryonic pharynx in the pharyngeal arches.
aplasia	Lack of development of a tissue or organ.
apoptosis	Programmed cell death.
atrophy	Degeneration of a tissue or organ.
bell stage	Tooth developmental stage at which the future crown is outlined as a bell.
bifid tongue	Cleft tongue, an anomaly of development.
blastocyst	Embryonic developmental stage forming a fluid-filled cyst.
blastomere	Early cell type produced by cleavage of the zygote.
bud stage	Initial stage of tooth development, budding from the dental lamina.
calvaria	Skullcap, the roof of the neurocranium.
cap stage	Tooth developmental stage at which the enamel organ forms a cap over the dental papilla.
caudal	Pertaining to the tail or tail region.
cervical loop	Looped margin of the enamel organ, outlining the future tooth root.
choana	Nasal opening.
chondocranium	Cartilaginous base of the embryonic and fetal skull.
chorion	The outermost fetal membrane, contributing to the placenta.
chromosome	The "colored body" of the nucleus of a cell composed of deoxyribonucleic acid (DNA).
cleft	Defect of facial and oral development; an abnormal fissure.
conceptus	Products of conception: the embryo and its membranes.
copula	Component of the embryonic tongue; conjunction of pharyngeal arches forming the posterior tongue.
cranial	Pertaining to the head or head region.
cyclopia	Condition in which there is only a single eye (in reality, fused eyes).

cytodifferentiation	Specialization of structure and function of embryonic cells.
dental lamina	Horseshoe-shaped epithelial band giving rise to the dental buds.
dental papilla	Formative organ of dentine; primordium of the dental pulp.
dentinogenesis	Process of dentine formation.
desmocranium	Embryonic membrane covering the brain; precursor of the skull.
diarthrosis	Movable joint.
diploid	Double set of chromosomes (2n).
dorsal	Toward the back.
ectoderm	Outermost of the three primary germ layers; forms the nervous system and the epidermis and its derivatives (hair, nails, enamel, skin glands).
ectomesenchyme	Tissue of the neural crest.
embryo	Portion of conceptus that forms the fetus prior to the 8th week.
enamel	Outermost layer of the dental crown.
endochondral	Bone type formed in cartilage.
endoderm	Innermost of the three primary germ layers; forms lining of the gut and its derivatives (salivary, thyroid, thymus, and parathyroid glands, pancreas and biliary system).
fertilization	Fusion of spermatozoa and ovum to form zygote.
fetus	Conceptus from 8 weeks until birth.
fontanelle	Membranous interbony interval in the calvaria.
forebrain	Rostral end of brain; prosencephalon.
foregut	Rostral third of embryonic gut.
frontonasal	Anlage of the upper and middle thirds of the facial prominence.
genetic	Relating to genes, inheritance, or ontogenesis.
genotype	Inherited genetic constitution.
gestation	Pregnancy.
haploid	Single set of chromosomes, normal in gametes (1n).
haversian bone	Compact bone with concentric lamellae around tubular channels.
Hensen's node	Precursor of primitive streak; organizing center.
Hertwig's sheath	Combined inner and outer dental enamel epithelia.
hindbrain	Caudal part of the brain; rhombencephalon.
hindgut	Caudal third of the embryonic gut.
histodifferentiation	Specialization of tissues into various types.
Hox; homeobox	Genes with conserved DNA sequences controlling development.
hyperplasia	Abnormal increase in cell numbers.
hypertrophy	Excessive enlargement of an organ or tissue.
hypoplasia	Underdevelopment of a tissue or organ.
incus	Middle-ear ossicle (Latin, anvil).
induction	Specific morphogenic occurrence influenced by an organizer.
intramembranous	Bone type formed in membrane.
intrauterine	Within the womb; refers to embryonic and fetal periods of life.
leptomeninges	Inner two layers of brain coverings (pia mater and arachnoid).
macroglossia	Tongue enlargement.
macrognathia	Enlarged jaws, particularly the mandible.
macrostomia	Enlarged mouth, particularly the rima oris.
malleus	Outer-ear ossicle (Latin, hammer).
mandibular prominence	Anlage of the lower third of the face.

maxillary prominence	Anlage of the middle third of the face.
Meckel's cartilage	Skeleton of the first pharyngeal arch; precursor of the mandible.
medial nasal prominence	Anlage of the central part of the face.
mesencephalon	Midbrain.
mesoderm	Middle layer of three primary germ layers; forms dermis, connective tissues, bone, cartilage, vessels, etc.
microglossia	Diminutive tongue.
micrognathia	Diminutive jaws, particularly the mandible.
midbrain	Central part of the brain.
midgut	Central part of the embryonic gut.
morula	Solid mass of blastomeres.
mutation	Transmissable alteration in genetic material.
naris	Nostril.
nasal fin	Transient embryonic membrane between the maxillary and medial nasal prominences.
neural crest	Secondary germ cell line arising bilaterally at the closure line of the embryonic neural groove; forms ectomesenchyme, the precursor of several tissue types.
neural plate	Specialized ectoderm that forms neural tissue.
neural tube	Anlage of the central nervous system.
neurocranium	Braincase composed of embryonic desmocranium and chondrocranium.
neurulation	Formation of the neural plate and neural tube.
notochord	Midline axis of the embryo.
odontoblast	Dentine-forming cell.
olfactory	Pertaining to the sense of smell.
oocyte	Female gamete prior to ovulation.
organizer	Agent or part causing differentiation or influencing induction.
oronasal membrane	Transient embryonic membrane between the stomodeum and the nasal cavities.
oropharyngeal membrane	Transient embryonic membrane between the stomodeum and the pharynx.
osteoblast	Bone-forming cell.
osteoclast	Bone-destroying cell.
osteocytes	Bone cells located in lacunae.
otic	Pertaining to the internal ear.
ovum	Female gamete after ovulation.
palate	Structure separating the mouth from the nose.
parenchyma	Functional tissue of an organ.
parotid	Largest salivary gland. Alongside the ear.
periodontal	Around the tooth; pertaining to the dental attachment apparatus.
pharyngeal arches	Series of paired arches in the embryonic neck region, demarcated by pharyngeal grooves.
pharyngeal grooves	Indentations of the embryonic neck region between the pharyngeal arches. The first groove forms the external acoustic meatus.
placode	Plaquelike thickening of ectoderm.

primitive streak	Initial germ disk axial organizer.
primordium	The first recognizable stage of embryonic development of a structure or organ.
prominence	Protrusion or swelling.
prosencephalon	Forebrain.
pulp	Innermost dental tissue.
Rathke's pouch	Stomodeal diverticulum; anlage of the adenohypophysis.
Reichert's cartilage	Skeleton of the second pharyngeal arch; anlage of hyoid, styloid, and stapes bones.
rest	Persistent fragment of embryonic tissue in the adult.
rhombencephalon	Hindbrain.
rostral	Toward the cephalic end of the body (Latin, beak).
somite	Segmental paired block of mesoderm; anlage of the vertebral column and segmented musculature.
somitomere	Rostral paired mass of partially segmented mesoderm; anlage of the cranial muscles.
spermatozoon	Male gamete.
stapes	Inner-ear ossicle. Also called the stirrup.
stomodeum	Midfacial ectodermal invagination; anlage of the mouth and nose.
stroma	Supporting framework of an organ.
suture	An immovable fibrous joint in the skull.
synarthrosis	Immovable joint between bones.
synchondrosis	Cartilaginous joint.
syndesmosis	Fibrous joint between bones; a suture.
syndrome	Consistent complex of symptoms and signs.
synostosis	Bony joint.
teratogen	Agent or factor that produces defective development.
teratology	Abnormal development.
trimester	Any of the three 3-month periods of gestation.
trisomy	Presence of an extra (third) chromosome in a diploid cell (2n + 1).
tuberculum	Eminence or swelling.
uterus	Womb.
ventral	Toward the front.
vestibule	Entrance to the oral cavity.
viscerocranium	Facial skeleton derived from the pharyngeal arches.
zygote	Fertilized ovum (from *zygos*, yoke)

INDEX

In this index, page numbers in *italics* designate figures; page numbers followed by "t" designate tables. *See also* cross-references designate related topics or more detailed topic breakdowns.